THE ULTIMATE MEMORY MANUAL

Learn How to Remember the Things You Used to Forget

JON NELSEN

Life Level Up, LLC

opinions or values of the company that individual works for or any others. Under no circumstances will any blame or legal responsibility be held against the publisher, or author, for any damages, reparation, or monetary loss due to the information or quotes contained within this book. Either directly or indirectly.

QUANTITY PURCHASES: Schools, companies, professional groups, clubs,

and other organizations may qualify for special terms when ordering quantities of this title.

For information, email info@jonnelsen.com

This book is printed in the United States of America.

<u>Also By The Author</u>

Nonfiction

What College Didn't Teach You About Getting Hired: The Ultimate Guide on How to Find a Job After Graduation

Planners and Journals

#1 Goal and Habit Daily Planner: Undated 90 Day Productivity Planner

The Little Black Beer Book: Tasting Journal

Interview Series

One More Beer, Please (Vol. 1): The Largest Collection of Interviews With Brewmasters and Craft Breweries in History

One More Beer, Please (Vol. 2): The Largest Collection of Interviews With Brewmasters and Craft Breweries in History

One More Beer, Please (Vol. 3): The Largest Collection of Interviews With Brewmasters and Craft Breweries in History

Introduction

> *You have brains in your head. You have feet in your shoes. You can steer yourself any direction you choose.*

~ Dr. Seuss

So before we dive into the meat of this book, let's talk about a few fundamental principles that everyone on this planet can relate to.

These principles can not only shape the way you live your life, but form the lens through which you view the world. I'm asking you to read these and truly comprehend what they mean, because simply grasping these concepts will be enough to change the trajectory of your life and perhaps your family's life decades into the future.

And rather than hearing these thoughts from me (you don't know me yet), I want you to hear it from people who have already made their impact on the world. An impact that perhaps you might still make as well…

<u>YOUR MINDSET IS YOUR ONLY LIMITATION</u>

> *I will not let anyone walk through my mind with their dirty feet.*

~ Mahatma Gandhi

> *The snake which cannot cast its skin has to die. As well the minds which are prevented from changing their opinions; they cease to be mind.*

~ Friedrich Nietzsche

> *Stop giving other people the power to control your happiness, your mind, and your life. If you don't take control of yourself and your own life, someone else is bound to try.*

~ Roy T. Bennett, The Light in the Heart

<u>LEARNING MASTERY HAS A METHOD</u>

> *If people knew how hard I had to work to gain my mastery, it would not seem so wonderful at all.*

~ Michelangelo Buonarroti

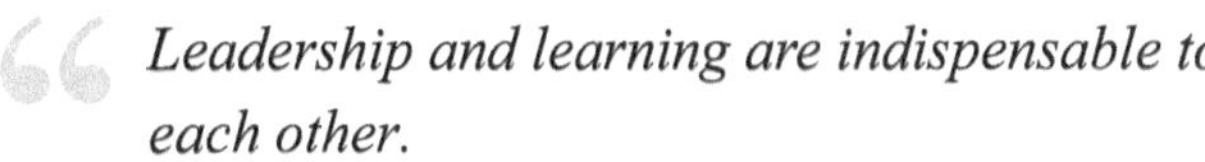

Leadership and learning are indispensable to each other.

~ John F. Kennedy

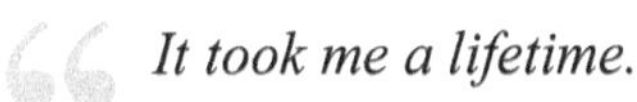

It took me a lifetime.

~ Pablo Picasso

THE BEST TIME TO MAKE A CHANGE IS RIGHT NOW

Everyone thinks of changing the world, but no one thinks of changing himself.

~ Leo Tolstoy

Yesterday I was clever, so I wanted to change the world. Today I am wise, so I am changing myself.

~ Rumi

Discipline is the bridge between goals and accomplishment.

~ Jim Rohn

If I have one singular goal through writing, it is to change the way people view themselves in the world around them. With this goal in mind each book is broken into three simple parts:

The Mindset

The Method
The Implementation

I do this because we live in a world that wants to make you small and take away your control. We're surrounded by people who want to tell us we're limited in what we can do, believe, or achieve. The worst part is if you don't learn to rewire your thinking, you can start to believe the nonsense and negativity.

Through mastery of your mindset you can train your brain to become your biggest asset and strongest ally. When you take the time to learn the best methods for accomplishing something, you increase your ability to achieve it exponentially. And finally, when you have learned enough to get started, it's time to take action. Implement the knowledge you have gained and start. Just start, don't wait, don't allow doubt to creep in, like Nike says, Just Do It!

I write each book to help you fully understand the most basic ideas of a concept and remove the illusion that rapid change takes dramatic effort.

- Life is a series of small steps and tiny victories.
- Decide who you are, what you believe in, then test why you have those beliefs.
- Decide what your goal is and make sure it matters to you on a deeper level.
- Visualize your achievement of the goal
- Then work BACKWARDS from that goal to where you are today. Create the steps, think about the obstacles, and make them so small and manageable that each day, week and month you are continuously marching towards your dreams.

I have written several books and I hope that this will be a lifelong effort demystifying the anxieties, worries, and stresses people maintain. There is no giant mystery to what I do, and I am not some uniquely gifted writer or philosophical thinker. I simply study the best advice and information available about a subject and distill it down into actionable pieces. Helping people just like you achieve what they want out of life by using a logical, systematic, and repeatable approach.

The keyword is ACTIONABLE, because you must choose to take action or you will never become who you want to be. For years I had the biggest dreams and the shortest attention span. I would aspire to greatness, but get overwhelmed by the process. It took a rewiring of my mindset to determine that breaking a goal into almost microscopic parts and achieving daily victories makes it easier to triumph than fail.

Why this book matters?

This book is about transforming your memory into a powerhouse that can easily reference the unlimited information around us. A great memory is one of the strongest ways to build your brain and achieve measurable success. We all know exactly what a strong memory will do for our lives, and I don't need to sell you on what you're missing. You already know your memory stinks and you're reading this because it's time to make a change and take back control. It's time to stop feeling like a victim of your mind's whimsies or distractions. So read on and I promise you I won't waste your time. You are about to read *The Ultimate Memory Manual* and I guarantee it will improve your life.

If you are the type of person who truly cares about reaching your potential and becoming the hero of your own story, visit me at: jonnelsen.com

Simply by visiting you will gain access to FREE books designed to build you up and resources to help you achieve maximum results for you life.

Good luck on the journey,

Jon Nelsen

Part One

THE MINDSET

 "Right now I'm having amnesia and déjà vu
at the same time. I think I've forgotten this
before."

— Steven Wright

Your memory sucks! That shouldn't come as a
surprise, right? At the critical moments when we
need to remember something, it fails us. When
we need to recall important information for a test or recite
data for our boss, it disappears faster than a magician. And
memory isn't simple, as some might think. It is a world of
study that even medical experts haven't yet fully under-
stood. It is a puzzle that even the greatest of philosophers
have not been able to decipher completely. Sometimes you
may wonder why some people can't remember even the
simplest things when it's critical. It could even be you,
letting everyone down at those crucial times because you

can't remember important facts when they count on you. Memory is just so vital to our everyday life that not using it properly can have a truly adverse effect on our well-being.

I USED to work as a bartender, and my memory was the worst. Oh, I could remember what beer someone ordered to drink 3 months ago, but ask me their name five minutes after hearing it, and I would draw a blank! Why is it that I could perfectly recall random pieces of information while missing the most critical parts? I hated that feeling like I was a complete idiot because I would forget things everyone else seemed to remember. Enough was enough. I decided that I would learn more about how the mind works, so I never again had to embarrass myself by asking for someone's name a 5th time.

BEFORE YOU DECIDE that trying to develop a better memory is a waste of time or not worth your effort, let me give you a few facts.

Your brain can remember more information than you can learn in a lifetime

ACCORDING to Northwestern University psychology professor Paul Reber, "If your brain worked like a digital video recorder in a television, 2.5 petabytes would be enough to hold three million hours of TV shows. You would have to leave the TV running continuously for more than 300 years to use up all that storage."

It has an incredible capacity to memorize and recall, that at just 11 years old, Nischal Narayanam claimed his first Guinness World Record—for most random objects memorized. (In case you want to beat it, he memorized 225 random objects and the numbers assigned to them in a little over 12 minutes.)

It is also worthy to note that the adult human brain can store trillions of bytes of data. As evaluated and concluded in a Stanford research, the cerebral cortex alone contains 125 trillion synapses. That's a whole lot of storage space, and before you get to start calculating, let me ease your stress—one synapse stores up to 4.7 bits of data. Ideally, 1 bit is equivalent to 1,000 bytes, and 1 trillion bytes equals 1 Terabyte. So if you multiply 125 trillion synapses with 4.7 trillion bits, then you see that the cerebral cortex alone has the capacity of storing around 74 Terabytes of data. Even an average 21st Century laptop can store enough information with a capacity of 1 Terabyte. This shows that your brain has the capacity to retain and remember any size of information.

A good memory will make you happier

DR. TRACY ALLOWAY, who led the research at the University of Stirling, carried out a study of 1,200 people aged from their late teens to their sixties. "We found that people who have a high working memory tend to be more optimistic, more hopeful about life, more confident that they can cope with problems and adjust to situations."

A faulty memory can lead to depression

IN THAT SAME STUDY, Dr. Alloway found that "People with a poor working memory tended to be more brooding and to spend more time fixated on problems when they arose in their life." In other words, more likely to become clinically depressed.

Simply closing your eyes really helps you remember better

LEGAL AND CRIMINAL PSYCHOLOGY found that, when people closed their eyes, they could answer 23 percent more questions correctly about a movie they had just watched.

How we lie matters

ACCORDING to research from Louisiana State University, false descriptions—elaborate inventions of the imagination—are easier to remember than false denials (when you deny something that is actually true).

Scientists still don't know if photographic memory can be learned or even exists

WHILE IT MAY NOT BE possible to train your brain to have a photographic memory, you can improve your memory through mnemonics and other techniques. Simple things like sleep and exercise also help boost memory.

The brain is like any other muscle; if you don't exercise your memory, you weaken it

INTEGRATEDLISTENING.COM REPORTS that "the notion that the brain can change in response to stimulation, an ability known as "neuroplasticity," is now so widely accepted it can be called fact. A pioneer of this groundbreaking idea, Dr. Norman Doidge describes how the brain can change in response to specific and repeated stimulation in his best-selling book on neuroplasticity. We can essentially re-wire it through specific and repeated input. As in building strength and endurance with physical exercise, we can build neurological pathways and synaptic activity at any age."

IF OUR HAPPINESS and success are tied to a healthy brain and we can grow it like any other muscle, why wouldn't we choose to develop an amazing memory?

IN THE NEXT CHAPTER, we will learn about the different types of memory and how to make them work to your advantage.

 "A clear conscience is the sure sign of a bad memory."

— Mark Twain

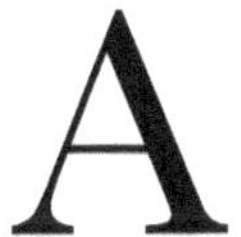s we tackle this topic, let's start with the basics.

What is Memory?

MEMORY IS NOT JUST REMEMBERING a particular thing in life; it's the process of retention. We keep information in our minds over time and turn it into past stories and events. Memory is the brain's function to retain information after the body's senses have processed it. It is such an important part of our personality that it literally helps define who we are and how the world relates to us.

Memory is so imperative, which is why losing the ability to remember things is one of people's biggest fears. Losing memory terrifies people in a way that only sharks and public speaking can. Yet, why does the brain lose its ability to remember? Why do we become so forgetful? Are there factors that trigger forgetfulness?

And while we view forgetting a memory as a problem, sometimes, it may be a necessity. Because of this, our mind categorizes our memory function into three specific types.

In Majid Fotuhi's book, "The Memory Cure: How to Protect Your Brain Against Memory Loss and Alzheimer's," he breaks down memory into three types; long-term memory, short-term memory, and procedural memory. Let's look at each and unravel the mystery of our minds.

Long-Term Memory

LONG-TERM MEMORY IS the one you've been keeping for years. Fotuhi explains that people remember a memory that's important in their history. We might not forget our wedding day ten years ago, but not have any clue what we were up to a month before that special day. He sets the example of the World Trade Center bombing on September 11, 2001. This is a notable event in America's history. On that morning, people can still remember everything they were doing. After knowing that they bombed the center, people cried and talked so much about it. The news spread around the world. People felt the impact of the bombing and couldn't take that moment off their minds.

MEANWHILE, they may not remember what happened on September 10, 2001. That's because the events that day weren't as notable as the ones the day after. I still remember exactly where I was on September 11th, but cannot remember much of what I did the rest of that year.

THINK of long-term memory as the brain's version of a bookmark. It won't always give you the context of the surrounding pages but will help you reference something that was meaningful or interesting. Learning to better harness our long-term memory is this book's goal.

Short-Term Memory

SHORT-TERM MEMORIES OCCUR when we memorize a detail
for a while and then forget about it. This kind of memory
is purposeful, so you memorize something only for a
specific purpose, i.e., an exam. After serving that purpose,
your brain will gradually forget it.

FOTUHI GIVES an example of a restaurant server. The server
needs to remember the order of every customer that comes
in. He might memorize many orders during a day, but all
of those stored orders will be forgotten by the time he
drinks his first beer after work.

I EXPERIENCED the opposite situation as a bartender. I
would store memories of drinks someone ordered and their
face in my long-term memory, yet I could easily forget
names and other important details relating to the experience. It was in learning more about how our brains worked
that I developed an interest in harnessing the memory
skills I knew I had for the purposes I wished.

Procedural Memory

LONG-TERM, short-term, what's next? Just like the name,
procedural memory functions 'procedurally.' For instance,
a particular dance routine for a competition. It stays in
your memory for weeks after the competition. The dance

doesn't leave your memory because you've adapted to the song and the routine.

Fotuhi said that this learning takes place in the cerebellum and basal ganglia. These are the parts of the brain that are good at learning new movements. Those who suffer terrible memory issues can often still operate on procedural memory.

This is something that you might see in a movie. Someone gets in a car crash, forgets their name and all details of their life, yet makes their coffee in the same way they always did before the crash. Procedural memory is the way you might drive to work and get there while still half asleep.

Encoding, Storage, and Retrieval

Now to take everything a step further, let's discuss how our mind works to retain what we learn and see in the world.

Encoding

THIS IS the all-important first step in the process of memory. Let's look at the two parts that make up a successful encoding of a memory:

• LEARNING OR PERCEIVING - This is simply the interaction you have that causes your mind to pause and take notice.

• RELATING to previous knowledge or events - This is where your mind references how this might be like something you discovered in the past.

LET'S go over a familiar real-world example and think back to our days in high school. Now I won't ask you to remember that embarrassing moment with the girl you had a crush on (we all know that's thankfully forever stored in our long-term memory); we are going to think back to our hardest science class. If you were a science wiz, maybe math or English was your tough class. For me, I was awful at chemistry, which was weird because I was a wiz at any science classes related to animals, the planet, and any typical earth science class.

WITH CHEMISTRY, things would go in one ear and out the other. The reason was that I struggled to draw on past reference points to help me understand and compare to previous knowledge. In my science classes that dealt with animals or plants, I had unlimited reference points in my head to visualize, categorize, and group what I was learning. To this day, I don't fully understand the difference between an Alkali metal or a Transition metal. Ask me what element number 72 Hf is, and I will look at you with a blank stare and punch you in the nose. Sure, it didn't help that I had no interest in those things, but not forming a relatable picture in my mind was the biggest reason for my struggles.

So if we know that the Encoding part is the most crucial in forming memories, we need to learn to form reference points to what we come into contact with. Learning to relate new experiences to past knowledge is the key to forming long-term memories of common everyday moments. As we will learn later in this book, it's not as difficult as you may think.

Storage

The next part of a memory we will discuss is Storage. If you think back, you will remember (hopefully) that we discussed that our mind is like a supercomputer able to hold the equivalent of 3 million TV episodes. So you know by now that storage is not an issue of our brain. In fact, I believe in the future, we will integrate memories into folders in our minds with the help of computer chips, but that is a story for another book. For now, we are just an organic group of cells with firing neurons that can store several lifetime's worth of data.

ACCURATE STORAGE of memories is critical and is one reason that witness testimonies are historically unreliable in the court of law. To store something for later reference, we need to make sure we accurately encode it first. We already know that we can store memories in our brain as either short-term, long-term, or procedural, and to remember something for life, it needs to become long-term.

Retrieval

LAST, retrieval is recalling the long-term stored memory from your mind. Retrieval is interesting because there are certain ways the brain has adapted to retrieve the information it has stored.

THE FIRST TYPE of retrieval we will discuss is Serial Recall. Basically, you might remember something as it relates to a series of events. For instance, you remember the next item in a recipe, but only after putting in the ingredient that proceeds it.

. . .

FREE RECALL IS another way we can retrieve information
that is random with a structured order. You might just
remember a piece of stored data in your brain and not need
anything to cue it up to make that happen. This is the best
type of memory to achieve, as it doesn't depend on
anything else to grab a memory we need.

ONE LAST WAY we might retrieve a memory is by priming
our brain to remember certain cues. We often refer to this
as Cued Recall, and it's secret memory champ have used
to remember the impossible. Are you familiar with the
work of Ivan Pavlov and his dogs?

THE BASIS of that study was that Pavlov trained dogs to
salivate in response to cues they associated with food. So
instead of a dog salivating because it was about to eat, it
would salivate when it heard a noise that meant food was
about to arrive. In the study, he used a metronome. I have
noticed this same response from dogs I've owned; when I
open a certain cabinet that contains their food.

WE CAN CUE our brain in much the same way. For
instance, say you wish to remember the veggies and fruit
that you need to buy at the grocery store for the week.
Rather than remember it as one comprehensive list
containing both, separating the list into veggies and fruit
could make it easier to remember.

. . .

In 1966, Endel Tulving and Zena Pearlstone conducted an experiment involving cued recall. Participants were asked to remember a series of words. In one group, they placed the words in categories such as furniture or professions. In the other group, the words weren't in any categories at all. The test results showed that the group who had cues (categories) remembered 75% of the words vs. 40% for the other group. The bottom line, Cued Recall, is very effective in helping you remember information.

"I can only note that the past is beautiful because one never realizes an emotion at the time. It expands later, and thus we don't have complete emotions about the present, only about the past."

— **Virginia Woolf**

Let's discuss all the problems that come with remembering and why we so often forget. We will focus on some common reasons why we have issues with remembering things.

ASIDE FROM SIMPLY AGING, there are many root causes of memory loss. We will tackle the actual problems that people have with remembering. Among the elderly, we often attribute memory issues to the degeneration of the body and age-related diseases like dementia and Alzheimer's disease.

HOWEVER, though many of us are young and have normal mental health, we still forget things, and here are some reasons:

Poor Retrieval

SOMETIMES you suddenly can't remember a memory or account of something.

THE FEELING that you know you remembered something, but that memory just vanished. We attribute this problem to the brain's poor retrieval of stored memory. It may be because of a lack of focus in remembering or an underlying symptom of something worse. Usually, it is because of a problem during encoding and can be easily remedied with a few simple tricks.

The Decay Theory

FORGETFULNESS IS a big reason people have challenges with remembering. A term known as the decay theory is used to explain the concept of poor recovery. The decay theory says that a chunk of memory "decays" when a person creates a new one. It is universally accepted that neurons die off slowly as we age, but some older memories may be stronger than more recent memories. Decay theory primarily concerns the short-term memory system, which suggests that older memories are often more shock-resistant or retained when there are physical attacks on the brain. Though the memory is in there somewhere, we bury it beneath recent memories we have added. Over time, that memory will disappear if there's no attempt to remember. Simply put, the decay theory says that you forget things you don't repeat or rehearse. The memory "decays" and later becomes forgotten.

Encouraged Forgetfulness or Suppression

PEOPLE GIVE 'INSPIRATIONAL' quotes and motivational speeches to a grieving or depressed person. But the person experiencing pain may want to forget those painful memories. I call this "encouraged forgetfulness." This concept entails that we encourage a person to forget their saddest experiences. It is a natural occurrence in a society that often struggles to deal with past sadness and pain. Any memory that adds to your 'worst moments' in life isn't an encouraging one. Many people tend to 'throw those memories away' so they don't brood over them.

AFTER A BREAK-UP, the death of a loved one, ill-luck, or failure on a critical school test, all you want to do is forget. You don't want to think about them so you can have peace of mind. The tendency to 'move on with life' and 'forget it ever happened' is one reason people forget. We even forget memories before or after the painful event. We try hard to ignore these memories, so we don't get overwhelmed with anxiety. Pain is exhausting and unkind and does so much harm to the heart and mind. So, of course, we often want to avoid the pain and fix ourselves.

ACCORDING TO SOME PSYCHOLOGISTS, consciously forgetting something painful is suppression. However, unconsciously forgetting a painful memory is repression. Not all psychologists accept the repression theory because of the challenges in studying repressed memory.

Interference

IN THE SAME manner that interference can jam up a signal on your radio; in psychology, interference can jumble up memories. Interference isn't a conscious effort to forget a memory but a result of mixing up two or more memories.

Two memories with similar events may get mixed up as your mind focuses on the 'most beautiful' or the 'most recent.' It's somehow filtering your thoughts and manufacturing memories; thus, it brings out a false memory.

Information Overload

THIS RESULTS from learning information and then immediately learning additional information after that. When that happens, it can make it difficult for our brain to keep what we just learned because it couldn't process the new information before we piled additional information on top. The best solution is to take breaks between new pieces of information. Much like a rest between sets at the gym, our minds need time to recharge before we continue learning additional material.

Forgetting old memories

MANY TIMES, we forget an old memory because we have new ones. The need to focus on 'the present' somehow comes to us unconsciously. We're living in the moment and trying to adapt to an unfamiliar environment, which leads to forgetting older memories.

Forgetting new memories

THE REVERSE CAN ALSO OCCUR; an old memory could just
be the one you'll remember rather than a new one. That is
because memories may be more powerful and relevant
to you.

THE NBC TV series "This Is Us" portrays Rebecca
Pearson as someone who forgets simple things like where
she kept her phone. But she remembers every moment of
her early motherhood days. Those times were more special
to her than the current times, which could happen with us
too. We could value older memories because those were
wonderful times.

LIKEWISE, Majid Fotuhi writes about a 1940 brain tumor
surgery that took place at the Montreal Neurological Institute in Canada. Brenda Milner, PhD., a Psychology professor, worked with Wilder Penfield, M.D., a neurosurgeon,
on the procedure. Dr. Milner observed that these patients
had problems with recalling or encoding fresh memories.
Yet, they could remember the oldest memories of their
lives.

THE PATIENTS who met and talked with her would forget
her when she left and came back only minutes later.

These patients would also repeatedly laugh at the same joke even after it is told three or four times. They'd laugh as if they'd never heard it before. This is also a problem of acquiring new information (Fotuhi). This was because of the surgery removing the hippocampus. It is a brain organ that helps with memory. So, if a person's hippocampus runs short of its function, that person could forget newer memories. But they'll be able to keep older ones.

Lack of Interest

SOME MEMORIES ARE MORE important than others, and we usually place a tag on that memory. When people like a particular thing, they attempt to remember it. But when a particular event is of no interest, there's no effort to store the memory. Interest comes with a particular person or thing that's significant in life. It's not your fault if you're not interested, but it also causes you to forget instances with some less than interesting people or events.

Passage of time (Transience)

WHEN TIME PASSES BY, memories fade away, and that's one reason we forget. We inevitably have to ignore one memory or the other because many events keep us busy. In

Psychology, they refer to this passage of time as "transience."

TIME PASSAGE CAUSES so many changes, and one of them is the ability to recall a specific memory. The average adult human can store about 2.5 million gigabytes of memory. However, what's weird is that sometimes the memory vanishes by the next day or week. After a year, it's excusable that you forget a memory, but forget something the next day? Some brain scientists insist that this memory problem is helpful. This is because the brain filters a flood of memories to highlight the few far more important ones. I tend not to agree; I like to remember everything.

Thinking too often

A PERSON who's an over-thinker on life's problem may struggle with forgetfulness as well. Thinking and analyzing is good, but it affects your memory a lot when you overthink particular subjects.

A DEPRESSED PERSON could suffer from memory issues. Forgetting because of being depressed could be harmful to your brain. If you're depressed and need to see a therapist, you can find one specializing in memory retrieval.

Misattribution (Failure to Recall Completely)

Now, some situations occur where a person loses the information meant for storage. This isn't usually intentional; instead, there's a failure to store the information in the brain. The memory never had the chance to stay in your mind, and with that, you've failed at recalling it. Sometimes, we aren't aware that memory has escaped from our thoughts. Little details like the color of a car could skip our minds. All we could remember is the size of the car. A chair of Harvard University's Psychology Department, Daniel Schacter, wrote a book called The Seven Sins of Memory: How the Mind Forgets and Remembers. He adds misattribution as one type of memory failure.

Sleep levels

According to a study from Harvard-based Nurses' by Howard Lewine, "too little sleep, and too much, affect the memory." The study showed that people deprived of sleep at night often have illnesses related to blood flow, reducing the brain's capability to store memories. Likewise, those who have too much sleep are forgetful as well.

.   .   .

So, not getting enough sleep can affect how you recall information. Your brain is tired and weak, and it needs some rest. It's easy to understand how poor sleep could deteriorate one's memory. But you may find it hard to understand how long hours of sleep would affect your memory. These people have "poor sleep quality" (Harvard Health). You must analyze how you can best manage your sleep to improve your productivity and recall.

Lack of attention

REMEMBERING IS AN ACT OF ENCODING, storing, and recalling information. Not paying attention could lead you to forget. If we don't focus on an activity, event, or people, the brain will not have enough time to encode it in its memory areas properly. As a result, when you're asked or need to remember an insignificant event in your life, you will most likely have forgotten it. An example is remembering what food you ate yesterday or the day before. If the food isn't that memorable, you will most likely forget it.

THERE IS one reason we have issues remembering that is more powerful than any other. This one issue can break the wills of even the strongest men and women. It can cause them never to reach their goals, dreams, or aspirations. In the next section, we will discuss the powers of belief and why it is the single most important factor in gaining control of your memory. Learning to harness your beliefs is the foundation for anything great you want to achieve in life. If you want the memory of a superhero chess master, the first step in controlling your thoughts and mind. Your ability to attain mindfulness gives you the complete edge over how your memory works and much concentration you can put in on vital activities that matter in your life.

Let me show you how to control your mind and thoughts in three simple steps:

Practice Mindful Meditation

Not everyone believes that this works anyway. At least a handful of people I've talked with made excuses for their being unable to concentrate. If you are one of such or have the thought about giving that as an excuse, then that's the first thing you need to eliminate from your thoughts; because that's not true. Meditation works. It is a process where you learn how to focus your mind on activities beyond your physical environment.

According to a study by Harvard researchers, it is believed that Meditation helps reduce stress, insomnia, increase productivity, reduce distraction, wellbeing, anxiety, worry, and enhance inner peace. If you want to learn how to master and control your emotions, thoughts, and minds, you should learn to meditate.

Weigh Your Thoughts

DON'T JUDGE; just observe. Not every thought in your head needs to be given total attention. Some need to be flushed away. Ever been on a project in the office, and over time you remember how you surfed the week before and how the waves helped your board peruse the ocean? Thoughts like this have no place in an environment like the office, especially when handling a serious project. What you need to do is observe and let it go. It is in the place of judging the thought and recalling how it all went that you become distracted. You need to be deliberate with your thought.

Create a Space to Align Your Thoughts and Mind

BY SAYING THIS, I meant that you need to your mind a clear path to align with your thoughts. That way, you are developing with Gerald Edelman called "the primary consciousness," which underlies all thoughts.

.   .   .

CLAUDE DEBUSSY's analogy makes clear sense in all ramification; according to the French composer, it is the "space between the notes that makes the music comprehensible." This implies that without space, the sounds wouldn't make sense at all. In this state of awareness, you empty your mind of wandering thoughts that you attain peace and total focus. Thus, until you attain this level of consciousness, it is very hard to control your mind.

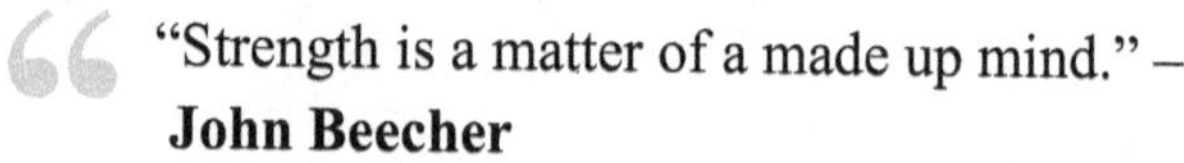

"Strength is a matter of a made up mind." –
John Beecher

As the title of this chapter says, we are now going to learn how to harness our minds to help us master our memory. I just as easily could have put the power of beliefs in the last chapter because there is nothing more detrimental to our growth than negative self-beliefs. However, just as the mind can work negatively to affect your performance, the opposite is true. Our minds are the most powerful muscle in our body and can power us to incredible achievements if we only learn to harness it. Before we talk about the positive power of our minds, let's discuss some negative self-beliefs that hold us back and where they come from.

. . .

Every day we are bombarded with advertisements and media that tell us we are incomplete or less than because we don't have this or have too much of that. And we can't be mad at the advertisers or companies, because they are just doing what they need to in order to sell a product. To make matters worse, marketing negativity is just the tip of the iceberg for our beliefs. They base some marketing on hope, but marketing experts learned long ago that fear of want or loss is the strongest motivator. We also have several other cracks in our tough exterior that allow negativity to creep in.

Self-defeating thoughts can stop our momentum before it even starts. We may have grown up in a household where family members put us down and told us we could never achieve our dreams. Perhaps it was "friends" who, rather than build you up, tore you down. Maybe you still have those "friends." Our internal pain and self-defeating mindset could come from many sources, but rather than focus on problems, let's focus on the solution.

Let's build our mind into a fortress with ever-expanding walls that continue to strengthen our belief in ourselves. Let's gain the tough mental mindset needed to achieve the ultimate memory.

We all know people who see the world as a constant struggle with the odds increasingly stacked against them.

Think about that person right now. Do things seem to go their way, or do their thoughts become a self-fulfilling prophecy? When I think of the stereotypical negative Nancy (Sorry to any Nancy's reading this) in my life, they never seem to have things go according to plan. They seem to fail before they start, and more often than not, rather than take personal responsibility, they blame problems on things ALWAYS outside of their control.

LIKEWISE, I know people who, despite tremendous obstacles, persevere and seem to turn problems into opportunities. The major difference between those types of people is often just their mindset and the things they believe. In order to have the mindset needed to achieve astonishing results with our memory, we need to start with the proper mentality. Let's begin with an important question to set the stage.

SO NOW THAT you know why you want to improve your memory let's talk about commonly held myths about our memory.

Myth 1

I wasn't born with an excellent memory, so I will always be forgetful.

THIS IS 100% false! We are born with exceptional memories, and it's the reason babies can absorb information like a sponge. From the moment they are born till about three years old, children have the most capacity to learn new things and remember them. However, that doesn't mean that because you grew up, then you're screwed. That just means you have to work harder and give yourself more opportunity to remember important things to you. Everyone was born with a tremendous capacity to remember details and information, and everyone can improve the memory that they currently have. Sure, you may never get in the Guinness Book of World Records for remembering the digits of pi, but you can learn to remember the names of everyone you meet.

Myth 2

My brain can only hold so much information; if I learn one thing, I forget another.

OUR MINDS CAN HOLD MORE information than the greatest supercomputers. That means that you could fit several lifetimes' worth of knowledge and information into your brain and still have room for more. Once you master the correct method of encoding, storage, and retrieval that works for you, you will draw on the information you surely would have forgotten years ago.

Myth 3

 Some people are blessed with photographic memories, but not me.

MOST SCIENTISTS AGREE that photographic memory does not exist. It's a popular name that someone made up, but it's not real. Yes, some people naturally have better memories than others. But that's the beauty of life; it doesn't make any difference in the world what other people can do. All that matters is that you improve yourself from where you were yesterday. In this life, the only person you are competing with is staring back at you in the mirror. Memory champs are not blessed with some superpower. They have naturally gifted minds that have been sharpened through 1000s of hours of practice and mnemonic devices. There have been many studies that have confirmed that the people with the best memories did not achieve their accolades simply by chance. They worked hard for years practicing their craft and learning every trick to master their mind. You can practice and learn everything they did!

Myth 4

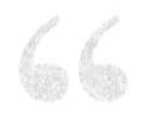 Memories are fixed and never change.

WE CAN ALTER memories without even trying. Yep, you can remember things one way, and after many years and external factors, we can alter memory in our head. Emotions you feel, and beliefs that you believe can affect previous memories stored in your head. It's up to us to guard against external and internal forces that can alter memory and make it less reliable. We will learn how to avoid misremembering later in this book.

Myth 5

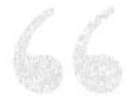 Your memory works like a video camera recording events for playback later.

THAT IS a simplified version of reality. Because we are living breathing creatures with emotions, dramas, traumas, physical and emotional changes our as we said before, our memories can develop slight alterations. That is normal, and the most important thing is that we learn to encode in a way where we prevent that from happening. Without a disciplined approach to your memory, it is quite possible that your mind's video recording isn't what the camera saw through the lens.

Myth 6

> If I don't learn visually, I can't have a powerful memory.

IT'S NOT what we see with our eyes that matters. It's what we see with our minds, how we visualize the information we're inundated with. The information we often retain the best is the information we see with more than just our eyes. The more senses you engage when encoding a memory, the better. Think of our senses as triggers. You might remember a cheesecake if you saw it across the room. However, if you smelled the sweet fragrance of fresh cheesecake, grabbed a fistful with your hand, and shoved the flavorful cool cheesecake in your mouth, you would have engaged more senses and thus improved your memory encoding of that moment. While you can't always engage all of your five senses during encoding, you can work to engage as many as possible. With practice, you can even try to trick your mind into engaging senses you didn't engage!

Now that we have dispelled various myths that the uneducated public believe about memory, let me bullet point a few things you need to understand and internalize.

• You were born with an exceptional memory, and the power to keep information is still inside you.

• Science says that memory is key to a happy life, so improved memory will make you happier.

• Once you commit to improving your memory, you will see improvements in areas you never expected.

• You will never fill your mind to the brim, so you can happily learn every moment of every day. Your mind can accommodate any level or capacity of information you give it.

• When you are about to learn something new and difficult, you can prime your brain to get ready. Much like a vaccine prepares us for a larger dose of a virus, a small exposure to something new prepares us to be ready to retain more information about it in the future.

• FAILURE IS nothing more than feedback. When you've inevitably forgotten something you vowed to remember, don't get down on yourself. Analyze why it happened and how you will try to avoid that outcome in the future. That way, you improve your mind with every positive AND negative outcome. This is something that separates the good from the great.

I HOPE you see the amazing opportunity that lies ahead of you. If you are excited to transform your life and strengthen not just your memory but your entire mind, it's time to commit to making it happen.

THE LAST CHAPTER of part 1 deals with discovering your WHY. Why you want to improve your memory, and what that will do for the rest of your life.

Why Do You Want to Improve Your Memory

 "A good snapshot keeps a moment from running away."

— **E. Welty**

While gaining a better memory comes with a host of benefits, it's not an easy task to achieve. As humans, we're naturally prone to forget. To solve the problem, we must first be aware of what we want to do - which is to have an incredible memory. Then dig deep to discover the motivation to make a change. We need to know what having a better memory will mean in our lives.

A BETTER MEMORY means that we will have more control over our lives. It will change the way we think about the world. It will develop our brain, focus, and ability to make wise decisions. Also, an enhanced memory will help you make that right decision quickly. We will better adapt to circumstances and work our way around problems and dilemmas with ease.

WHATEVER FIELD in life we find ourselves in, a better memory is beneficial. A better memory will change our personal, social, emotional, academic, and professional lives.

Personal Life

A BETTER MEMORY will help you become better as a person. You can fuse all the meaningful memories in your life to help you keep composure in times of emergencies.

SOMETIMES YOU NEED to progress in your career, your attitude, and your mindset. With an excellent memory, these things could fall right in place. A better memory helps to manage your life plans and helps you learn lessons from history. It also helps us weave a rich tapestry from our past full of memories we hope never to forget and moments that make us smile. Memories connect moment to moment and give us chances to see progress, growth, and change linearly.

Helps to Manage Plans

When an excellent idea pops up, and you later remember it, you can make plans for it. A good memory helps you remember those aspects of your life that you can change and what moves to make.

In the next chapter of this book, you'll learn how to develop your memory. That way, you'll figure out how to manage plans properly.

Learning Lessons From History

Mistakes we've made in the past guide us through the future. The saying goes, "we learn from our mistakes." But if you don't remember your mistakes, would you learn then?

Memories of mistakes pain us, but it can help move forward, avoiding the same mistakes. Sometimes, we need to remember our past mistakes to keep our bearings in place and not get sidetracked again by failures.

. . .

WITH BETTER CONTROL over your memory, you can store crucial memories from the past. Sometimes good and sometimes bad, remembering the past help inform our future. It is especially so if you know how to cope with negative memories and use them to enhance your present and future lives.

Improves Creativity

A BETTER MEMORY improves your creativity as much as it allows you to make the right decisions. Many times, creative people adopt ideas they've seen somewhere else. So, remembering those ideas would trigger your creativity. The world's filled with creative concepts that others make that can be repurposed to help us conquer projects and opportunities. It makes you think of innovative ways to work on something new.

Social Life

HAVING BETTER memories can help you improve your social life. At events, social gatherings, and parties, your keen memory can avoid awkward situations like forgetting someone's face after talking to them or not remembering people's names. Social interaction will be more efficient, as you will remember most of the conversation you will make with people.

When you remember faces, you can increase your social circle of acquaintances. That's because, like in social interaction, the conversation flows. The inability to identify a person's face is called prosopagnosia. You aren't able to encode the structure of the person's face enough to recognize them later. That could be awkward when that person meets you elsewhere.

Being Better at Love

Having a better memory can lead to a better love life. Remembering key details that will make your love life better is important. Many breakups result from forgetfulness, and it's a real thing. The worst part is that a forgotten memory often becomes a memory your partner will NEVER forget. Learning past mistakes is one way that a better memory can affect your emotional life. Or it might be as simple as remembering you made dinner plans and showing up on time. Either way, an excellent memory will make a big difference to someone special.

Academic Life

We all know that they created schools for the learning of formal subjects you might never need. But what if it turns out the things we learn might help us in our future if we can only remember them? Remembering and understanding lessons are at the forefront of every school's goal. Remember the lessons, duties, and all the things that determine your grades in school. A good memory will apply all lessons taught and improve on it for a practical exam. Best of all, it might prove applicable to your future!

Being More Intelligent

When you have better memory as an academic, you're able to connect different theories and ideas. You aren't limited to a particular topic because you have a broad knowledge of many things in that subject. Remembering doesn't merely give you good grades. You're also able to have a more intelligent mind that captures so many ideas.

In class, you could even be more inquisitive when you're divided into groups. You're also able to ask your Professor intelligent questions where necessary. Many times, people who cram don't get the best grades. But people who genuinely understand a topic are those who get the A's. That's because they aren't working with the short-term memory where they have to memorize a lesson. They can transfer what they learned to medium and long-term memory. This comes with the bonus of ACTUALLY learning something for the future as well.

Being More Reliable

HAVING A BETTER memory doesn't stop at getting A's or being the most intelligent person in the class. Whenever you're serious about your academics, your Professors would recommend you to anyone. Also, they'll have confidence in you for anything. And that's because you have such a sharp memory.

THERE'S nothing better than a group of people who believe in you, especially if those people might help you in the future because you showed an aptitude for the subject when others struggled to remember it.

Better Stage Presence

THERE ARE some lessons in school that require an audience, and once you have a wonderful memory, it'll be easy for you. Many people claim to have stage fright during a

speech presentation or stage recital. This is because of
"being afraid of forgetting." While other people might fear
the number of people, you may just be afraid of forgetting
your lines. That happens a lot. When you've mastered your
memory, you're able to remember all the points to consider
during the speech. Your confidence matters, but excellent
recall will boost that confidence!

Learning New Concepts in Class

HAVING A BETTER memory will give you the ability to
learn new concepts in school. Paula Fiet, a student
researcher at Weber State University, discovered that
short-term memory is why many students have problems
learning unfamiliar concepts in the classroom. Many
students don't understand concepts in Maths, Physics,
Literature, and Geography. They can't keep hold of the
information, even though the teacher has explained it
several times.

SHE ADDS that you need working memory to learn these
unfamiliar concepts. She also says, "Children with poor
working memories don't get enough information in their
minds to make sense of what is coming in." It means that
those referred to as 'slow learners' in class have a challenge with their memory. That's why many parents
embrace homeschooling or private tutoring for their chil-

dren. They need to be always reminded about these lessons, but what if the child's memory fails? It's best to work on your memory so you can adapt to learning new concepts.

Professional Life

BELIEVE IT OR NOT, remembering also improves your professional life. Just imagine what a better memory would mean at your workplace and with your clients. Remembering key facts, figures, and obstacles will help your boss notice the next time a promotion is coming up.

Better Focus

SOMETIMES AT WORK, there's a pile of tasks awaiting you, and all you have to do is to focus. Connecting details is vital in the work environment. The average workday pulls us in so many directions; it's easy to lose sight of vital goals and timelines. A better memory will allow you to concentrate better on your tasks at work. You won't lose track of all the work you should get done.

. . .

WITH BETTER FOCUS, you can also figure out how to use equipment you haven't used before. Sometimes, we learn new things at work. It's up to us to solve the puzzle, and remembering experiences can help. For instance, you're using tables in your Word document. You would need to insert an Excel spreadsheet into it. You understand that there could be an option to insert the Excel spreadsheet. And perhaps you only remember that because you learned it during a computer class in middle school. Imagine the time you would save by being able to recall that information.

A BETTER MEMORY helps you to be creative. It also contributes innovative ideas to work. It will impress your team with your efforts to make the company advanced. It shows you are dependable, and that is what every company looks for in a future CEO.

Lower Dependence on Machines That Sometimes Fail

WE ALL KNOW that technology is most likely to fail when we truly need it. Even in this Wi-Fi connected world we live in, there will be times when you simply need to remember. There will be a time when you can't access your saved notes or calendar, and in those moments, your memory is all that stands between you and failure.

. . .

IMAGINE the typical phone assistant we all have on our smartphones. You set a to-do list just in case you 'don't remember.' Then you remember this task about a week later, and you check your to-do list. Your digital assistant didn't remind you of anything! That's a technology failure. As humans, once we have improved our memory, we won't have to depend on apps that aren't reliable every time.

Solving Problems

SOLVING problems becomes more natural when the original pieces of the puzzle make sense. The world's connected, and it's up to us to see how one thing affects another. The people who can spot the connections and remember them when it counts are the ones who solve the problems and change the world.

Cognitive Development

APART FROM SCHOOLWORK OR LECTURES, having a better memory has a positive impact on your brain. How intelligent can you be? With a powerful memory, you can answer questions and analyze situations intelligently and instantly.

WHEN YOUR BRAIN KEEPS INFORMATION, it makes you
smart in every way. You can present an argument and
defend it because you remember pertinent facts. That way,
you aren't "arguing blindly."

Challenges the Brain

GIVING your brain some routine memory tasks can help to
challenge it. With a better memory, you're able to think
better. As we age, the more we exercise the brain, the
longer we stay sharp. Working the brain's memory muscle
is the best way to slow down the natural decline and stay
sharp in the years where you need it most.

Agile Brain

YOUR BRAIN BECOMES active when the memory is in good
shape. Neurologists claim that remembering many old
facts makes your brain responsive. We call this state
"mental gymnastics." It's almost like your brain is flexible
and can do all the neurological stunts, just as gymnasts do.

. . .

HAVING an excellent memory allows your brain to get used to working healthily. As it becomes a habit, your brain could save you in many situations. The National Institute of Health and Aging has several reports from memory research. The reports found that adults who had some memory training have more active brains than those who didn't. Also, after five years, their brain activities continued to stay active.

BEING a person with better memory is fantastic for every reason you could think of. You have so many areas of your life that you need to apply that memory. With good recollection, you can work better, study better, and sleep better. Analyze all the benefits that a better memory offers you. Decide if you want to do what it takes to train your brain.

Why Do You Want to Improve Your Memory?

BEFORE THE GREATEST progress and biggest transformations, we need to reach that point of no return. That is the power of programs like AA; people don't join them when their partying makes them feel like they're on top of the world. Nope, people join AA when they reach rock bottom, and it is only then that they have the strength and courage to change their future. You see that strength comes from a negative place but has positive results.

.   .   .

LET'S think about why we want to improve our memory in much the same way. What is it you have missed out on because of your sucky memory? How many memories of irreplaceable moments with your children are lost simply because you don't know the right way to tuck that memory into your mind? How many details from the first kiss with a spouse or last moments with a beloved relative have been lost to the oblivion of our unfocused brain? Whatever moments and opportunities passed you by because you couldn't remember, that is your reason, and that is your why!

When your reason WHY is stronger than your fears of a full commitment to improvement, that is when you are truly ready to grow...

Now, just imagine the opportunities at work simply by better remembering the names of people you meet. Imagine walking into a room with people who you haven't seen since last year's trade convention and greeting them all by name. You think that might make an impression? Or what if you could store and keep key details about watching your son pitch his first little league game? Imagine the joy that would bring you holding onto that cherished memory in old age. What if you were on the verge of another argument with your wife, and instead of fighting, you recall with pinpoint accuracy the moment you first met and remind her of it? Do you think she will still want to throw that frying pan at your head then?

It's easy to make light of all the amazing things we might gain from a powerful memory, but the results are real. We know that it will allow us to avoid unforeseen consequences that result from poor memory. Similarly, we can only guess what gifts a stronger memory might hold in store for us. Take a moment to make the decision that you will commit to change and won't rest until you improve your memory!

In any drastic change, the most important part is establishing WHY you want to improve. The HOW is only a small portion of the equation; it's the WHY that's needed to arrive at the solution.

Before we learn exactly how experts remember in Part Two, make sure you have firmly established why change is so crucial to your life. Without deciding to commit to a new you, it will be difficult to focus and drive to improve. So take a moment and do this before we move on.

Part Two

THE METHOD

Stuffing Your Face for Maximum Memory

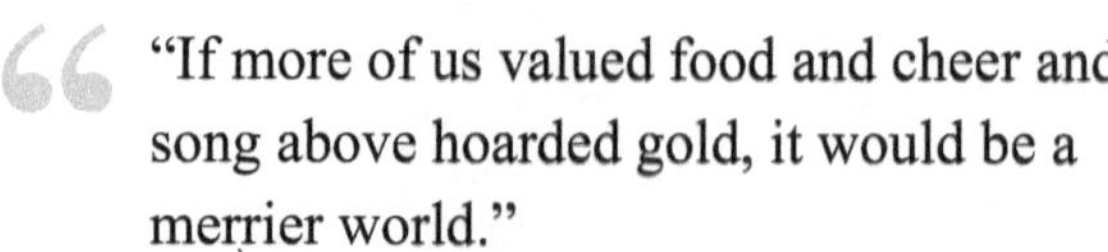

"If more of us valued food and cheer and song above hoarded gold, it would be a merrier world."

— **J.R.R. Tolkien**

Did you know that the foods you eat can help your mind gain focus, clarity, and improved memorization? Simply incorporating some of these basic foods into our diet is one simple way to build that memory muscle. Since so much of improving your memory is mentally taxing, it's great to know that some things take almost no effort.

Here is a list of the best foods for memory

I will remind you I am not a doctor, so consult a licensed physician before making any dietary or medical changes.

• **Fatty Fish** - Seafood like trout and salmon are amazing memory boosters. The reason is because our minds are made of fat tissue, and a good portion of that tissue contains Omega-3. Omega-3's found in much of the seafood we eat, and it is one of the building blocks of our minds. According to Martha Clare Morris, who studied the effects of fish consumption on the brain, they even believe that the omega-3 found in fatty fish can help ward off Alzheimer's disease.

• **Coffee** - I'm pretty sure I heard a collective sigh of relief at the mention of improving memory with coffee. Many of us start our day with coffee, and it's the combination of caffeine and antioxidants that seem to help the brain the most. And according to Dr. Astrid Nehlig, coffee also has positive effects on a few neurological diseases.

• **Blueberries** - Come on, it doesn't get much easier than this. Simply pop a few blueberries in your mouth and enjoy the anti-inflammatory, antioxidant, memory-boosting goodness of nature's candy.

• **Turmeric** - One of the active ingredients in turmeric is curcumin. Like blueberries, it is a potent anti-inflammatory and antioxidant. Healthline.com also points out that it's an anti-depressant.

• **BROCCOLI** - This delightful green veggie is full of vitamin K, which helps the brain and is linked to improved memory. Along with vitamin K and a list of other great vitamins, it contains antioxidants.

• **PUMPKIN SEEDS** - Ever eat baked pumpkin seeds in the fall when you are carving pumpkins? As a child, I did, and little did I know that's probably the reason I can't ever forget the embarrassing moments I suffered in my youth. Like most everything else on this list, pumpkin seeds contain powerful antioxidants. In addition, they also contain significant magnesium, iron, copper, and zinc.

• **CHOCOLATE** - GOT YOUR ATTENTION, didn't I? It's specifically DARK chocolate that improves memory. But between you and me, I'm sure regular chocolate has some brain-boosting chemicals in there somewhere, too, right? When reading the ingredients of a dark chocolate bar, if you see it 65% cacao, all that means is that 65% of the weight's derived from cocoa beans (cocoa butter and cocoa powder also are included in that %)—basically, the higher, the better with chocolate content. Trust me; I lived in the sweet chocolate town of Hershey, PA, for much of my life!

. . .

• **NUTS** - THESE HAVE the double whammy of improving both your heart and your brain. Nuts are full of healthy fats, vitamins, and antioxidants.

• **ORANGES** - I'M sure you knew oranges were full of vitamin C, but do you know why that matters? Because, among its many benefits, vitamin C protects your brain from decline as you age.

• **EGGS** - ACCORDING TO HEALTHLINE.COM, "Eggs are a rich source of several B vitamins and choline, which are important for proper brain functioning and development, and regulating mood."

• **TEA** - No, I'm not talking about the iced tea you see at the gas station next to the milk. Real teas like green, rosemary, ginkgo biloba, ginseng, peppermint, and many others are tools in your fight for brain healthiness and memory improvement.

• **WHOLE GRAINS** - The last food on this list is whole grains. Because it's a rich vitamin E source, whole grains should be part of a balanced diet to help keep you sharp throughout your life.

. . .

THIS IS NOT a complete list of foods that will help your cognitive abilities and brain functions, but eating these will definitely get you going in the right direction. There are hundreds of different things you can eat that will help you gain an edge, but as long as you are getting enough antioxidants, vitamins (B, C, D, K), magnesium, zinc, or omega-3, just to name a few, you'll be just fine.

NOW ALL FOODS aren't equal, and there are certain things that should be shunned when trying to keep your brain in fighting shape. These items are not just bad for your mind, but bad for your body as well.

• SUGAR - THIS INCLUDES the sweets you love to indulge in, along with sugary drinks. Sodas, juices, and sugary sports drinks all cause your blood sugar and insulin levels to spike, impairing brain function.

• REFINED CARBS **and Processed Foods** - In the 1970s, before the action movies and the politics, Arnold Schwarzenegger was just a really freaking strong dude. He was the first truly global superstar bodybuilder, and if there was one food group he detested, it was refined carbs. He once referred to refined carbs as "White Death." What did he mean by that? Basically, all the white stuff (white rice, white bread, white pasta, white flour, and white sugar) is something you should abstain from if you wanted to perform optimally. Well, everything old is new again, and we are now more aware than ever that processed foods are detrimental to our health. The fewer chemicals and more natural you can eat, obviously the better. Those refined carbs do nothing to help your brain and therefore do nothing to help your memory. So "steer clear!"

• FAKE SUGAR - If it's made in a lab and you don't need to put it in your body, I wouldn't. Plus, fake soda tastes gross anyway; just drink water.

• ALCOHOL - I KNOW, this one breaks my heart too and is probably the sole reason I'm not on the New York Times Bestseller list. On a serious note, I'm pretty sure no one thinks drinking alcohol will do anything good for their body, but now you can't say I didn't warn you.

Author Notes -

Just so you know, I'm not an alcohol killjoy; I interviewed hundreds of American craft breweries about all things craft beer and created the largest collection of brewery interviews in history. I have been told it make a great bathroom book...

Check out: One More Beer, Please!

Not everyone will understand, but the bottom line is, what you put in your body really makes a difference in how well you function, most importantly, how your memory works. Your brain consumes more than a 5th of your body's total energy, so optimal nutrition will yield optimal performance. If you're serious about mental retention, your diet shouldn't be taken lightly. You need to make sure your brain is at its best always by feeding it the nutrition.

Habits Matter

> "Your beliefs become your thoughts,
>
> Your thoughts become your words,
>
> Your words become your actions,
>
> Your actions become your habits,
>
> Your habits become your values,
>
> Your values become your destiny."
>
> **— Gandhi**

So if you made it this far, you have committed to transforming your mind no matter how difficult it might first appear. We also spent a little time reviewing what should and shouldn't be part of a brain-boosting diet. We are still in the foundational stage of memory improvement. This chapter will discuss the everyday habits that affect our memories.

ONCE WE MASTER the control of these everyday habits, we will be ready to learn the fundamental techniques for memory improvement. Exciting, right? We haven't even gotten to the meat of this book yet, and you already have a better grasp of what it takes to achieve elite memory than 95% of the population.

NOW I WILL NOT ASK you to rearrange all the habits in your life, just a few. Shifting our habits is one straightforward way of preparing ourselves for the change about to come.

Don't: Multitask

THE FIRST BONEHEADED habit we have in our lives is the idea that multitasking works. I know it doesn't, you know it doesn't, and countless scientific experiments have proved it doesn't, so why do we keep doing it? My theory is that it is a way to relax our brain.

THINK ABOUT IT, if we don't give full concentration to the task at hand, doesn't it feel easier? By giving a little effort here and a bit of effort there, we do not force ourselves to focus and concentrate on one task. I know when I try to multitask; I move half as slowly and accomplish a third as much. Humans are not designed for efficient multitasking.

So instead of tricking your mind into thinking you are some amazing multitasking superhero, FOCUS on the specific task at hand. You already learned that true mastery of memory requires stimulation of multiple senses in a single event. If you learned nothing else in this book, I would challenge you to eliminate the idea of multitasking from life.

Do: Activate Your Senses with Purpose

Let's go back to the hypothetical memory of our son's baseball game. During a typical baseball game, most times, you are probably texting, answering emails, or playing Tetris on your phone, right? Heck, I do those things when I'm sitting five rows behind home plate at a Yankees game; it's just human nature. But the difference is, I don't need to remember that moment. I don't even like the Yankees, and baseball can get boring! You need to remember your son's game, and you need to keep this memory, or you will regret it. Here's how:

. . .

• **LOOK** - Don't take your eyes off the field for 5 minutes. Look at every detail, the dirt on the uniforms, the color of the grass, the faded sign in the outfield, the right fielder picking his nose. Treat this moment like a buffet for your eyes; you are taking a mental video of this moment.

• **TOUCH** - Stay still, just for a moment. Don't fidget or move your body at all. After you have calmed the movement of your body, start slowly fidgeting to engage the Haptic memory. Touch the bleachers you are sitting on, or slowly feel the denim fibers of your jeans. Whatever you want to do, stick with that specific fidget. One singular type of touch can help us carry this memory into the future.

• **SMELL** - Jordan Gaines Lewis wrote an interesting article in Psychology Today about how smell affects our ability to remember. She said, "Incoming smells are first processed by the olfactory, which starts inside the nose and runs along the bottom of the brain. The olfactory bulb directly connects to two brain areas that are strongly implicated in emotion and memory: the amygdala and hippocampus. Interestingly, visual, auditory (sound), and tactile (touch) information do not pass through these brain areas. This may be why olfaction (smell), more than any other sense, is so successful at triggering emotions and memories."

· · ·

THEREFORE, memory is so often tied to what we smell. To this day, I can smell freshly baked bread and be taken back to my grandma's kitchen. As I'm sure you have experienced in your life, the smell is one of the best ways to conjure up vivid memory.

WE CAN USE that to our advantage while trying to remember this little league game too. Take a few deep breaths and try to smell the freshly cut grass and bowl of halftime orange slices. If you can do it without looking like a weirdo, smell the leather of your son's glove when you are walking back to the car. Anyone who ever played baseball knows there's not another smell like it.

• **TASTE** - THIS IS one of the most difficult senses to activate in any practical sense. Like smell, taste can trigger retrieval clues of a memory. The problem is, we only taste so many things. One of the best ways to use this to your advantage is to eat or chew something relatively unfamiliar during encoding. You would then repeat the eating or chewing during the retrieval of that memory. Next time you are studying for an exam, pop some weird flavored gum into your mouth and chew that same flavor during the exam itself.

• **SOUND** - SCIENCE HAS UNFORTUNATELY NOT YET CAUGHT up to my opinion, but lucky for you, I will still present it and let you decide. We have not yet proven that music itself will help you remember, but we know it does a few important things that may help. First, listening to music changes our mood. That means if you put on something that relaxes you and makes you happy, you might be more receptive to new stimuli making memories. Second, our brain's wired in such a way that we sometimes use the left side or the right side more depending on the cognition required for an activity. When we listen to music, we can activate both sides of our brain. Again this is my assumption, but until proven wrong, I believe that the more of our brain that's activated during a memory, the easier it will be to recall that in the future.

DURING YOUR BASEBALL GAME, you might really focus on the sound of the ball hitting the catcher's glove. Or perhaps you can better store the crack of a wooden bat from a left-field hit. Either way, pay attention to the surrounding sounds, especially ones that are situation-specific.

ACTIVATING our senses is just one trick we can use to help increase our memory retention. This is a habit that requires extra effort but gets easier and more natural with repeated practice.

Do: Congratulate Yourself When You Remember

WE OFTEN BEAT ourselves up when we make a mistake and don't take the time to congratulate ourselves when we succeed. Try to catch yourself being successful and reframe your mind. Limit the moments you allow yourself to feel disappointed in what you did or didn't do and relish the moments where you made yourself proud. Each night try to reflect on the many wins you experienced throughout the day. Often without this reflection, these accomplishments are simply swept under the carpet of our minds.

Do: Remember Why This Matters

FROM TIME TO TIME, it's important to reflect upon what this means to our life. Remind yourself why you so desperately want to improve your memory. Continue to be hungry to learn and excited about improvements. Stay motivated and work to get just a little better each day. Over time, these incremental daily improvements will become large personal achievements.

Don't: Worry Be Happy

AS THE SAYING GOES, "Don't Worry, Be Happy." When we relax, we are the most open to our surroundings. All that worrying takes energy and effort in your mind. Rather than stress about things you might not have control over, try to find purposeful moments each day, week, and month where you recharge and refresh. A clear mind is a powerful tool.

Do: Always Be Present

THIS IS a habit that I struggle with the most, yet it is the one that is most important. For many, including myself, it is a daily battle to be in the moment and not dwell on the past or worry about the future. Being in the moment naturally reframes our thoughts to spot the things we are missing. It helps us activate more senses without effort, and in a general sense, allows us to be happier.

LIVING in the moment will allow you to look back and have memories rather than regrets. If you are always concentrating on what's next, you miss out on what's now! When you want to focus and plan for the future, do it purposely. Don't take away from the active moments happening around you to worry about what's coming. Likewise, don't sit there daydreaming about the wonderful times in the past and miss out on the incredible beauty in front of your eyes. There is always another time to plan or reminisce, but you will never get right now back. ALWAYS BE PRESENT.

Do: Exercise

Everyone already knows that exercise is good for you, so I won't belabor this point. For brain health and memory, exercise does a few key things that everyone will see a major benefit from. First, it increases oxygen to the brain, which helps the brain function at 100%. Also, it reduces the risk of multiple memory loss disorders and diseases. Exercise causes your body to release positive chemicals like dopamine and endorphins to the brain. Those are the feel-good chemicals that make us feel like we are floating on clouds and overall improve our disposition. But that's not all. Exercise also helps your brain remove the chemicals that cause stress and anxiety.

So I know that exercise isn't something you wanted me to list for some people, but for the sake of your brain health, it might be time to get off the couch. If you are new to exercise, consult your doctor, and start small. Sometimes just going for a short walk is enough to make a significant difference in your body and mind.

There you have it, all the habits to build and break for memory. Get started today; don't waste any time. Even just being conscious of the things we are doing and not doing is powerful. Small daily habit tweaks can have a profound effect on your mind. Focus on small habits and everyday moments. Don't beat yourself up with failures but concentrate on your successes. It takes a lifetime of effort to build better habits, but the payoff is worth it. You can do it, just believe you can.

 "Every man's memory is his private
literature."

— Aldous Huxley

So before we move on to more advanced memory techniques, let's go over some easier memory techniques that have proven effective for generations. Mnemonic devices are still useful in this time and age to help you remember things. The only thing is that you have to create them for yourself or figure them out by yourself. It's often someone else that has created it, but you'll adapt to it for easy remembrance.

THESE DEVICES COULD COME AS ACRONYMS, phrases, rhymes, or songs. These are all related to the information that you want to remember. You could form a notable acronym that can make you remember easily. Or you could use the tune to your favorite song to trace all the information that you need.

Types of Mnemonic devices

MNEMONIC DEVICES ARE easy methods of getting that memory stuck in your head for a very long time. Other mnemonic devices include visualization, songs, the location method (method of loci), etc. Here they all are:

Acronyms

ACRONYMS and Weird Expressions

ACRONYMS ARE another great way to remember simple to complex bits of information. If you need to remember something critical and recall it with great precision, try this method. One method I use is that I will write every detail I need to remember on flashcards with the word on one side and a first letter of the word on the other side. I then lay them out in order and make the weirdest phrase I can, filling out a word that uses the letter on each card. Once I am done, I simply read the front and back of the card together several times, then place them in order and easily encode it in my brain. An example of this mnemonic device in action is the SWOT analysis or the common method of learning colors of the rainbow. How it works is that the initial letters of every item would form something notable.

EXAMPLE 1

AN EXAMPLE IS the SWOT analysis used in the business world to help employers and employees quickly. SWOT stands for Strengths, Weaknesses, Opportunities, and Threats (SWOT). We attribute the SWOT to Albert Humphrey, who created this mnemonic to show the things that need to be remembered and the importance of each word. 'Strengths' and 'weaknesses' come first in the acronym because they're internal factors. Meanwhile, 'opportunities' and 'threats' come second because they're external factors. This makes it easy to identify and analyze whenever they are at a conference. The person won't be caught unaware if asked about the SWOT analysis.

EXAMPLE 2

ANOTHER EXAMPLE IS the academic world. We all remember the 4th grade Visual Arts topic, "Colors of the Rainbow." Our teachers used a general mnemonic device that took over the globe, and it was also an acronym. It was "ROYGBIV" (Red, Orange, Yellow, Green, Blue, Indigo, Violet). This mnemonic device was inspired by Sir Isaac Newton's light experiment, "Roy G. Biv." It fits into the arrangement of the rainbow colors. With this inspiration, it has become fixed into the Color Wheel of Visual Arts Education.

Visualization

Everything visual is always something noteworthy. That isn't an overstatement. Many researchers have proven that visual information is the easiest to remember. Even when it's coupled alongside audio information, it gets better. Our brain enjoys visuals. It is familiar with the recognition of sounds and words when we view and review images.

As a mnemonic device, we can capture the information in our thoughts, so we create mental pictures—the more outlandish and memorable, the better.

Music

Do you remember how you learned the alphabet? Probably not, because it was so so long ago. But I would wager, if you start at A end at Z, chances are you will turn it into a song before you finish. Learning through music was fundamental to learning at a young age and is how the alphabet has been taught in schools for the last century. However, just because you are no longer a child does not mean that turning important memories into songs won't work to help you remember.

NEXT TIME you have important facts, figures, or dates that you need to recall, consider turning them into a song. As we already learned, music triggers multiple parts of our brain and can help us better encode and later retrieve information.

Rhyming

SIMILAR TO MUSIC and equally effective are rhymes. To this day, when I think of the days in a month, I will rhyme it in my mind. In school, we learned rhymes for presidents, states, and capitals with impressive effect. There will be other memory devices we learn later in this book, but for simple recall, it doesn't get much easier than creating rhymes.

HOOK MEMORY SYSTEM

THIS METHOD USES numbers and mental objects to trigger memories and keep the information fresh. This method works best for a smaller number of items that need to be recalled. To use this method, you would start by creating your hook system. To do that, you would number 1-10, and for each number, you pick an object that rhymes with it. An example might be one = Ton (a one-ton weight), Two = PU (something stinking), Three = Ski. After that, you have to form a vivid mental picture of those images in your mind as detailed as possible. So for Three = Ski, I would color the skis and designs on them. In fact, I might even envision a skier using them. Then say your numbers a few times out loud while picturing the vivid image. Finally, picture whatever you need to remember interacting with those images in order. So if you remembered to pick up baked beans, bananas, and orange juice at the grocery store, you could use this method.

I WOULD SIMPLY PICTURE a giant can of baked beans on a scale weighing a ton. Then a pile of stinky brown bananas with flies buzzing around. Last, a carton of OJ doing black diamond ski jumps in the snow. You can remember as many items as possible in numeric order by building those images in your head.

THIS IS one of my least favorite ways to remember something, but it is very effective for some people. I will encourage you to research this method if it seems like something that might work for you.

.   .   .

Chunking

THERE'S A SAYING THAT GOES, "if you want it big, start small." With this mnemonic device, you must break down a large piece of information into a smaller one. The purpose of this is to understand and encode the message easier. It's like reading a guide on "how to wash your car." You wouldn't have to memorize all the information written if it was a long stream of words. However, if you chunk it by applying a step-by-step process, the instructions will be remembered easily.

ANOTHER EXCELLENT CHUNKING example is the U.S. phone number. The U.S. phone number comprises 10 digits, designed to be chunked. You wouldn't memorize the number as XXXXXXXXX. Memorize it in three sets: XXX-XXX-XXXX. In fact, the phone number system used in the U.S. was specifically designed, so it would be easier for people to remember.

WHICH MNEMONIC DEVICE do you love the most? Try to identify the technique you'll be more comfortable using, and that way, you can solve your memory problems.

Basic Memory Tips

- Your brain is wild and can be unpredictable, and so we need to be the same. When you want to remember anything, be it a name, number, place, or anything else, make it strange in your brain. Say I need to remember the number, 1,475. To fix that firmly in my mind, I would picture that number as a giant fleshy statue, then imagine slithering snakes going through those numbers and biting it, so it was in a pool of purple alien blood! Yep, make it weird, and you will give yourself a better chance of remembering what you need to.

- I used to better remember names by associating the sound of a name with an image. So if I met a man named Brock, I would picture a big rock on the side of a cliff. This also works when you can connect the name to someone with the same name who is famous or you know. If I meet a man named Victor, I would picture Victor Frankenstein, and then, of course, I would think of the big ugly monster and boom, I will never forget my new friend Victor again!

- Continue to engage the senses when you want to remember. So once again, with Victor, I would imagine the loud ARRRHHHH Frankenstein makes and the putrid odor of a creature made from pieces of dead bodies. Whatever senses you are trying to engage, give your mind time to visualize and "feel" it. At first, you will be slow, and the memory process will feel laborious, but as you continue to practice, you will get faster and more efficient.

• • •

• WRITE IT DOWN! When you want to memorize something, write it down on paper. Don't type it on the computer, because there is something about pen to paper that helps our mind remember something effectively.

• CREATE a mind map to organize your thoughts. This is where your central idea will have multiple parts of a web with other similar ideas. I use this when writing a book. I picture what the principal topic is in my mind, and then the chapters become connected bubbles that I visualize as if I wrote them on a blackboard.

• REVISIT THE THINGS you wish to remember. Unless we reinforce what we wish to remember, our mind naturally experiences exponential memory loss. Not that we will completely forget what we are trying to remember, but the percentage of information we keep will slowly decrease. One simple way to counter that is to review what you learned. Begin by reviewing each day, and if you are finding the information sticks, you can space it out further and further apart. The key is tracking how well you remember what you need to and shortening the length between review sessions if you find out you forget details easily.

• • •

• TEACHING SOMEONE IS a great way to activate new areas of our brain and improve retention. If you want to remember a specific subject, try to explain it to a friend or your spouse as if you are a teacher. This will force you to organize your thoughts, and often the simple process of organizing those thoughts in our head protect us from forgetting.

THESE ARE JUST some simple ways to remember that may or may not work for you. Try them out, see which methods make sense for you and which you don't really care for. Everyone is different, and our minds are all unique. There is never a right and wrong way to remember, so don't get discouraged and just keep practicing. In the next chapter, we are going to learn more advanced methods of memory.

The Memory Palace

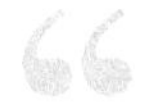 "Time's the thief of memory"

— Stephen King, The Gunslinger

Many believe this to be the single most powerful memory technique ever invented. This is an Ancient Greek/Roman memory strategy that has been used by chess grandmasters and memory champions. It's time to learn "The Memory Palace," and once you learn how to properly build your "palace," it will allow you to remember an unlimited amount of data.

A MEMORY PALACE is also referred to as "the method of loci, wherein "Loci" is Latin for "locations." It's a method used to recall information that a person has encoded. The Memory Palace is a mental location where you store images using mnemonic devices. As we already discussed, mnemonic devices are strategies you adopt to help you remember both simple and complex information.

While creating a Memory Palace, you go on a journey to a place that you're familiar with. There is a sequence that the journey follows. It is through that sequence that you're able to create your palace.

The Memory Palace helps you know how good you are at remembering people, places, and entities. It's not a physical palace, but it's a place in your brain where you store things from your memory. Also, it isn't so different from your memory. But it's a different concept, which implies that you want those memories stored. You create a Memory Palace based on places or things that you're familiar with.

History of the Memory Palace

We can trace the existence of the memory palace to ancient Greek history. People needed to have techniques used for retaining information. The writing materials weren't as natural to gain access to as in modern times.

. . .

THOUGH THE GREEKS invented the memory palace, it soon traveled throughout the world and was also discovered by the Romans. In his rhetoric, Cicero talked about the technique. The name of the rhetoric was "De Oratore." Cicero explained that the Memory Palace came from Simonides, a Greek poet.

SIMONIDES'S USE of the memory palace came from an event in his life. Simonides was invited to recite a poem for a banquet for the upper-class members of his society. After doing so, he left the event before it was over. Unfortunately, moments after he left, the banquet hall collapsed, killing everyone inside.

THE COLLAPSE WAS SO terrible that nobody could identify the dead inside the rubble. The only person who could identify the dead was Simonides. He remembered the location of each person was sitting in the hall while reciting. He noted where they sat, and when he went back to the position that he was in, he could start spotting them out. So, through this experience, Simonides created the Memory Palace technique because it worked! (Bower 1970)

IN ROME, the memory palace was very common. This is because of the fantastic results that its techniques brought to the people. The use and success in the ancient Roman empire have influenced many generations, which is the reason for its adoption even in recent times.

Dominic O'Brien is an eight-time world memory champion known for memorizing fifty-four decks of cards in order, that's 2,808 cards. He memorized it by viewing every card and what order they were arranged in the deck. Thomas Harris, a novelist, also mentions the Memory Palace in his novel, Hannibal. The character, Hannibal Lecter, uses the Memory Palace to locate patient records. His purpose was to track down people to kill.

How Does the Memory Palace Work?

The first thing to do while building a memory palace is to focus. If there's no focus, then there's no Memory Palace. Another thing that you must know is that you shouldn't be scared to focus. You may think it's a lot of work, but it will help exercise your brain as you create your memory palace.

The Ultimate Mnemonic Device

THIS METHOD COULD WORK WELL with your house, school, office, car, or anything you know well. When you use your mind to place objects in some familiar locations, you'd remember them. People even build a palace from scratch in their minds, but the trick is to create such vivid details that you become intimately familiar with the location.

Becoming a Good Memory Palace Creator Using Other Strategies

ASIDE FROM MNEMONIC DEVICES, there are other techniques you can use to become a Memory Palace creator. Many of these approaches are straightforward and make sense when you think about how they might apply to memory.

Have a technology recess

YES, sometimes take a break from technological reminders. Your brain may even work faster than technology. For instance, you probably have an app you use on your phone to remind you of things you often forget. You might have set an activity for a particular time. But if you can remember that event two hours ahead, it's more productive than an assistant. We rarely know what will happen in the next minute. I'm sure everyone has dealt with the power going out or your phone dying when you are expecting the alarm to wake you up for work. The same can happen when you always count on technology to make up for poor memory. Eventually, it will let you down, and it may be at the worst time.

IT'S BETTER to take precautions when trying to get a wonderful memory.

YOUR DIGITAL ASSISTANT doesn't help your brain. It only helps you with the next activity you have on your sched-ule, and that's all. You become so dependent on that assistant that your memory isn't challenged anymore. While you work on activating your brain, keep your phone or computer aside (except if you need it for work). This helps you concentrate on your brain and not on other elements around you.

Be Intentional

WHEN YOU NEED to recall something or someone, you have a reason to do it. If you genuinely want to remember, talk to yourself and say, "I have to remember this. I don't want to forget". Many times, speaking words to yourself provides positive results. And that's because you've set your mind to it.

. . .

AFTER MEETING A NEW PERSON, try using a mnemonic device to remember. For instance, the new person at your music school is "Samantha." You can remember the famous singer, Sam Smith. "Sam" with a "th" = Samantha. It's difficult to remember names, but when you need that person's name, you just have to go for it! Make the name interesting sounding or add details other than just the name. This was a technique former president George W. Bush used to memorize names and was displayed in the movie W. by actor Josh Brolin.

LIKEWISE, after visiting a place, create a reason you need to remember it again. Use some mnemonic devices to remember the name so you can recall it later on. This reason may not be valid, but you're only using it to develop your brain to remember things better. Challenge your mind never to forget this information every time you encode it.

BECOME Interested

YOU'RE TRYING to have a better memory, right? Why don't you try as much as possible to become interested? Becoming interested in a fact or idea helps you focus and remember easily. Sometimes, you won't need a mnemonic device. Your understanding of the information covers whatever distraction might make you forget.

. . .

Have it in mind that "this is a relevant subject." It may seem as if you won't need it anywhere you go. But in the long run, a conversation about it could spark up. You'll be able to contribute to it based on what you discovered by yourself.

Here is a prime example. Imagine you are watching a documentary about solar power in another part of the world. Knowing that your household doesn't use it, you may not be interested in remembering the key details. But if you can change your frame of mind, you can make almost anything more interesting. Instead, you decide to be interested because, soon enough, policies may change. Soon enough, perhaps developing renewable technology might become something that gives you a tax break and saves you money. Try to find an edge to make things more interesting and applicable to your life. In this example, when trying to boost your memory by becoming interested in solar, you won't think of using it. Instead, you'll tell yourself, "this is some interesting, safe technology. Let me know how it works". When you watch, you pay attention and spark your interest. It may even inspire you to check the internet for information about something new.

Take notes

This is the most common form of improving one's memory or 'remembering' something. When you need to remember a place, person, or thing, you write that information down. Writing it in your journal helps you to refer to it every time that you need the information.

FROM TIME TO TIME, you can write the information on a piece of paper. You need to ensure that it doesn't get lost. You should also not write all the information down. Preferably, write the chunks of information into your journal or paper. This helps to reduce the details of the critical points that you need for the information.

THE MOST IMPORTANT part of mastering the memory palace is concentration. You need to take the time to build out every detail in your head and make sure you can visualize your palace, so it's as detailed as looking at a picture in front of you. Once you truly master this, you will be among the most elite in the world of memory. The reason this is so rare is because of the initial difficulty. However, once you have an excellent strategy for building your palace, you will see how much easier this becomes.

> "Memories, even your most precious ones,
> fade surprisingly quickly. But I don't go
> along with that. The memories I value most, I
> don't ever see them fading."

— Kazuo Ishiguro, Never Let Me Go

Creating a Memory Palace is imaginary, yes. But it requires a detailed plan. You need to work with your brain for your memory development to be successful. It's a fun process and gets easier in time. Like many things, the first time you do it is the hardest, and after that, it gets much less difficult. You'll figure out you've been having a great time all along, and it's not as stressful as you thought it was.

Six Steps to Creating a Memory Palace

1. Select Your Palace

THE PALACE that you're selecting should be a place that you know well. The goal is to figure out how effectively the technique would work. You'll test your ability to identify things within that space that you've chosen as your palace. You should mentally be in that location, be it your home or office. With the technique, you're using your' mind's eye'.

FOR MORE EFFECTIVENESS, try using your home as your palace because it's the first place that you know. As you visualize your location, you're able to train your memory. Try to remember every object inside your room and visualize it in your head. You can either memorize it one by one or use the location method.

WHEN YOU REMEMBER the order in which they appear or where they are located, it helps you build your memory. Other palaces you can use include the streets, your school, your office, or a nearby park. It must be something you know well and can create a vivid image of in your head.

2. Identify Features

. . .

NEXT, you must note the parts of your chosen palace. If you picked your neighborhood, the first noticeable item would be the trash can at the side of the road. Now, walk mentally around your Memory Palace. Suppose someone jogging just threw a bottle into the trash can next to your home. What are the houses opposite the trash can? Also, what are their colors? If there are trees outside a particular home, whose home is it? Figure out that thing that captivates you—something that you can never forget. While remembering all these, take notes of them. Separate these items so you can fill them with the information you want to store in your memory.

3. Plan the Route

THIS STEP IS CRUCIAL. To create a memory palace, you need to plan out a map. For instance, you're using your school. There are so many routes that would lead you to different classrooms. Likewise, when entering your home, you may stop by at your brother's room before going into yours. So, be consistent with your route and follow it in your memory palace. Choose the path you prefer so it can be easier for you. So, if your school is your memory palace, record it to memory. Remember that you want to go straight to your classroom from the entrance. You can visit your school physically to follow the route. That way, you can remember how it'll appear in your Memory Palace.

. . .

I. YOU COULD MOVE from the school entrance to the exterior passageway.

II. Next, you go to the main door

III. Then the hallway.

IV. You move to the first staircase and then the second. Then you step through the first three doors on the right before getting to your classroom door.

YOU COULD EXTEND your palace to your seat in the class. Note that while walking and memorizing this route, you need to have a piece of paper. You need to write the typical features of each location. List visual features like color, material, size, surface feel, design, and shape. What does it smell like? The more of your five senses you can incorporate, the stronger the memory will be. The next time you try to run through the palace in your mind, you could try focusing more on the visuals this time and nothing else. Read through the notes you've taken and memorized the route. As soon as you're convinced that your Memory Palace route is set in your brain, you're ready for the next step.

4. Associate

. . .

RELATE an item you want to remember. Make it associated with the locations in your Memory Palace. You can take one piece at a time to make this process easier. Next, create a mental picture of these items and allow them to interact with your location. So, let's use the Memory Palace in the previous step—your school.

5. Start Using Your Mnemonic Devices

YOU ALREADY KNOW your palace and the route that you want to follow. You're also familiar with its features. You're now ready to use your mnemonic devices. Combine the use of a song, rhyme, or acronym to remember the information.

6. Revisit Your Palace

IT'S ALWAYS a great idea to revisit your palace. Go over everything that you've created. Ensure that nothing changed. But if you have, visit that change and ensure that it has already become a part of your Memory Palace.

THE MEMORY PALACE creation is always fun. It's exciting for everyone who uses it to improve memory. All that's required is hard work upfront to set your mind to a specific task, but you can develop almost superhuman memory. It exercises your brain and prepares you for challenging situations. This skill helps to boost your memory to the upper echelons of the brain's capabilities.

YOUR LIST WILL REMAIN in your memory for a few days or weeks. You can create more Memory Palaces for other things that you need to remember. They could come in different forms, and they don't need to be like the first palace you created. You can check the mnemonic devices list and the various loci you can use for your Memory Palace. If you want to, you can use the new loci, but be sure that you know the new loci structures before using them. Start by creating and dramatizing the scenario.

Tips on Creating a Memory Palace

CREATING a Memory Palace may seem difficult for you at first. Here are some tips for you to follow when creating a Memory Palace to make it a bit easier.

GETTING MORE loci

. . .

Locus is a particular point, position, or place, and loci are the plural form of it.

When you feel that you've used up all your loci with your other Memory Palaces, find another. For example, you can use the corner of your bed cabinet as one locus. The route will start from one edge of the bed cabinet and end on the other side. Other loci could include the right corner, the left corner, the adjacent wall, the opposite wall, the ceiling, the floor, and the entrance.

Your new loci can also be your friend's home or a video game map that you're familiar with. It can also be any other route that you're familiar with. Your favorite store, personal salon, gym, spa, shopping complex, and recreational park could serve as your loci.

Keeping Track of Your Memory Palace: Adding Qualities and Telling a Story

To keep track of your Memory Palace, you can write the journey and the several loci you'll use. You may also want to use the same locus at some point. What you should do is to add qualities to that journey.

. . .

ANOTHER WAY TO keep track of your Memory Palace is to connect items and your journey. That way, you're telling a story, which adds more ways to trigger a memory. You should create an account with your Memory Palace. Not only will it be fun, but you also can easily see the correlation between the items and your Memory Palace.

TAKE note that if the items are more than the loci, you can place two or three things in one locus. Ensure that these items can easily interact in that locus for easy remembrance. That way, your items aren't only relating to the loci, but they're also referring to one another. An example could be your Keurig coffee maker and the little cups that go in it. They interact together, but they're both used for different purposes.

SO, with the Memory Palace, you've told a story that has a plot (sequential arrangement of events), setting (your palace and loci), character, action, props, and light (well, not every locus should have such bright light, but that's a distinctive feature).

MEMORIZING a Short Book With a Memory Palace

TO MEMORIZE a book with your Memory Palace, you must first decide what you want to memorize. Is it the story?

The section headings? Or is it the entire text? However you want to do it, let's get started!

THE FIRST THING TO create is the palace. You should select your palace based on the locations we've discussed before. If your book has ten sections, ensure that your palace has about ten loci in it. That could be ten houses on the street or ten mailboxes at the houses. While you follow these directions, go over the procedures on creating a memory palace earlier in this book.

NEXT, start reading each section of the book. Once you're through with one, decide what you want to memorize from that section and fix it into the palace. Start your journey with the first chapter interacting with the first loci. You're reading a novel, for instance. You need to memorize each chapter for school or a research paper. Fit the chapters into your palace, and allow your palace to represent the entire book. The first chapter could be about a boy who lost his bicycle in front of a Haunted House. So what you do is to allow this action to interact with your first locus.

WHEN YOU GET to other sections or chapters, do the same. That way, you are tilting the story towards your immediate environment. It's almost as if you're bringing the story 'home' and not letting it die in the novel's setting.

. . .

So, if you're reading a self-help book, gather the lessons or concepts for each chapter. Let it associate with your loci. Likewise, if you're reading a novel or short story, allow the significant tale to relate to the loci in each chapter.

Changing Your Direction

Your locus has different directions, so you can change your direction if you want to be dynamic. For instance, your palace is at your house. You started your journey by walking towards the trash can and to the left of the road. Your new journey can have you move away from the trash can. It could begin with you walking to the right side of your lawn towards your neighbor's house. That way, you see an alternative view of the palace—different colors and designs, and various items around. You aren't only changing your direction, but you're also improving your point of view.

Overcoming Background Problems

It might be a problem if two of your loci have a similar background. And if your brain is using the background to recall information, that may be a challenge. It's better for you not to zoom into the color of the wall or the floor. This way, you can differentiate between the left wall and the right wall or the remaining floor corner and the right floor corner, respectively.

A REAL-LIFE EXAMPLE of the Effects of a Memory Palace

ONE THING TO know is that the Memory Palace is useful if you commit yourself to it. It also has nothing to do with your age, background, education, sex, marital status, or health condition. Anyone can practice it. Don't be discouraged if it is difficult as you start; it gets easier. Begin with remembering small things and work your way up to more complex memorization.

IN 2010, there was a study in Norway on how effective the Memory Palace could be (Engvig et al. 2010). Some experts trained 23 volunteers on how to use the Memory Palace technique. They were all about 61 years old. Each volunteer successfully memorized 30 words in the proper sequence within 10 minutes.

ANOTHER SET of volunteers of similar age, educational background, and sex were all a part of the study. They weren't trained in the Memory Palace Technique but were asked to memorize that list of 30 items.

.   .   .

THE RESEARCHERS ASKED the two groups to go on with their daily activities for eight weeks. After that time was up, the researchers asked what they had memorized two months before.

THE OUTCOME

AFTER EIGHT WEEKS, the researchers did something somewhat different this time around. They flashed 15 words unrelated to the trained and untrained volunteers. After which, they showed them 30 unfamiliar words. Half of the 30 words were unique, while they had displayed the others the first time.

THEY WERE all instructed to pick out all the words in the first 15 and call them in the correct order. The volunteers who knew the Memory Palace technique performed better than those who didn't. (Engvig et al., 2010).

ALSO, they could identify the correct positions of each word. They probably used mnemonic devices to support their memory. From the research, it's clear that the Memory Palace technique works for both long and short-term memories.

Part Three

THE IMPLEMENTATION

"If you wish to forget anything on the spot, make a note that this thing is to be remembered."

— **Edgar Allan Poe**

You have now have learned more about the methods and skills of memory retention than 99% of the population. This isn't the words of some author trying to hype you up; let's just look back at the knowledge you've gained just by reading this far.

YOU HAVE LEARNED the distinct memory types and what each entails:

• LONG-TERM

• **Short-Term**

• **Procedural**

NEXT, you learned the process of memory:

• **Encoding**

• **Storage**

• **Retrieval**

NOW IN AND OF THEMSELVES, nothing there is ground-breaking, but let's look at what that means to your life. You can now decide where you want to store a memory because you know the different memory types. Do you want it to be long-term or short-term? You can pick. Because you learned about encoding a memory, you know, to spend more time, focus, and review on something you want to remember permanently. You know why! Equally important, you can give less of your focus and effort to things that may only need short-term or procedural retrieval.

SPEAKING OF STORAGE AND RETRIEVAL, you know that you can easily store and later retrieve a memory if you activate more senses. How powerful is that? Without even expelling extra effort, you can activate additional parts of your brain by triggering your senses to help you remember.

See, the book paid for itself right there! But let's move on and go over a few other tidbits of knowledge I dropped on your head.

HOPEFULLY, you dug deep and decided that an improved memory would have a lasting positive impact on your life and was worth the struggle. You decided that you would cast away self-doubt and believe in yourself. Our beliefs are powerful and can be the catalyst to accomplish things we never thought we could before. You made a choice to believe in yourself and your ability to gain a terrific memory. I mean, you learned that a better memory = happiness and has a positive effect on every aspect of your life. Who wouldn't want to better recall people they met or one-of-a-lifetime trips they enjoyed? A better memory is a no-brainer…pun intended.

WITH A FEW SIMPLE tweaks to your diet and poof, your brain is supercharged and ready for knowledge. I didn't even rattle off a list of nasty vitamins and minerals you need to put in an older person's pillbox and take each morning either. Literally, it's as easy as eating more blueberries and dark chocolate. Maybe avoid a hot dog or two and any other processed food you were overindulging in and supercharge the process. At this point, your brain is getting the nutrition it needs, and if you remove some processed foods, your waistline will probably thank you too.

. . .

Don't forget the exercise! Get your feel-good chemical fix without the expense and hassle of a drug dealer. Dopamine and endorphins will make your brain feel good while simultaneously removing the chemicals, causing stress and anxiety. Plus, the added oxygen that exercise sends to your brain will help it function at peak performance.

You learned a few simple mnemonic devices that will set you apart from all those still using paper lists like dorks. Well, I guess you are still writing things down too, but only to commit it to memory, not to reference at the grocery store. There was a collection of tips and tricks to help you remember things in fresh ways, but the common denominator was creating a strong visual image in your mind. Doing that triggers a new area in your brain, which, as we know, will help that memory stick in there like super glue.

Finally, you learned about the mother of all mnemonic devices. The Memory Palace has been used for centuries to help people remember with precision and clarity that they thought it unnatural. As with every amazing thing in this life, it's not without cost. To really perfect, this skill takes time, training, and discipline. However, once mastered, you will have a superhero like mastery over memory. You can impress everyone with your ability to recall, and unless you compete in national memory championships, you might never meet your equal.

. . .

BE PROUD, you made it far in this book, and you really learned something. It's not always easy to get through something that's designed to teach you an incredibly complicated subject. In the next few chapters, we will go over the last keys to transforming your mind from what it was into what it could be.

Why Discipline Is Key to Results

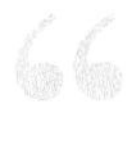 "I think it is all a matter of love; the more you love a memory the stronger and stranger it becomes"

— Vladimir Nabokov

There is and only ever was one thing that stands between you and everything you always wanted. It's discipline. If you were hoping I might say something else; then I'm sorry to disappoint. Building a powerful memory requires you to take a disciplined and intentional approach. You need to enter every single day seeking ways to practice and improve your mind.

NEVER FORGET that your mind is a muscle, just like your biceps or your quads. It needs to be worked, stimulated, and rested again and again. Today's world memory champions didn't get to where they are overnight. They trained and trained, determined to build their memory no matter how long it took or how difficult it was.

MY GUESS IS that you're probably not interested in becoming the next memory champ. You probably just want to improve the simple things in your life, like remembering someone you just met or not forgetting the bananas at the grocery store. That's ok; everyone is different, and so are the goals we have. But just because your goals are smaller doesn't mean that you're off the hook. You will still need to find simple ways to train your brain daily. To get the results you are looking for, you MUST be intentional. This isn't for the faint of heart or lazy. You will need to challenge your brain daily, and sometimes you will fail.

IN THE NEXT CHAPTER, we are going to discuss how to train our brains for success. If done correctly, you might find that you gain more than just a terrific memory. It's possible that through simple memory training combined with giving your brain what it needs to perform optimally, you will reach new heights with your career, friendships, family, and relationships. Proper diet and exercise can help your brain work harder, faster, and longer. Heck, if all this book taught you was what you needed to be quicker on your feet with comebacks, it was worth it. Discipline starts with putting yourself in the best position to succeed, so I challenge you to make the dietary changes needed to improve. Start exercising, even if limited, and build from there. Believe in who you are and what you could be. Once everything else is in place, it's time for training, and in the next chapter, I will show you just how to do it.

 "Memory is more indelible than ink."

— **Anita Loos**

Are you ready for some glorious news? Training your memory isn't as hard as it might sound. Sure, a few training methods require large amounts of concentration and effort, but most are pretty easy. I will start with a list of methods that are easiest to implement and the most fun.

BOARD GAMES

YEP, sometimes boosting your memory and cognitive ability is as easy as a weekly game night with your friends. Strategic thinking and decision making can activate different parts of your brain and improve cognitive skills. Best of all, if you steer clear of games involving Boardwalk and Park Place, board games decrease stress and promote happiness. They also improve patience and improve long and short-term goal setting.

Jigsaw Puzzles

SIMILAR TO BOARD GAMES, puzzles are another straightforward way to stay sharp and improve memory. A jigsaw puzzle's simple nature lends itself to effortless memory improvement because it forces you to use spatial memory. Spatial memory falls into both short and long-term memory and allows one to recall the different locations of objects along with their "spatial" distance to one another.

Improve Vocabulary

LEARNING and using unfamiliar words is also a fairly simple way to train your brain. You could get yourself a word of the day calendar and try to incorporate the new word each day. Supercharge this idea by both saying it and writing it down multiple times throughout the day. Vocabulary improvement is a simple way to get smarter, sound smarter, and feel smarter.

. . .

FIND an activity that will allow you to activate multiple senses at once. Go on a hike with a friend while taking the time to stop and smell the fresh mountain air. Join a cooking class and learn a new skill while tasting, smelling, and cooking. Walk around a flower shop and stop to smell the roses. All those activities are helping to give your brain a workout while also making fun dates. And if your anything like me, it doesn't hurt that a few of those dates are cheap too.

LISTEN to Music and Move your Body

LISTENING to music while dancing activates a ton of areas within your brain. We know that music uses both parts of our brain, and dancing incorporates our fine motor skills. And don't worry, even if you think your motor skills aren't that fine while you're moving on the dance floor, you can always dance in your room. It doesn't matter what you listen to or how you move, but the simple act of both will give your brain a boost in both power and creative thinking. What to be a triple threat? Add in singing to the music while dancing, and you will work your brain like a memory champ and feel like NSYNC. Add that to your daily routine, and you can say Bye, Bye, Bye to brain fog once and for all.

· · ·

Change Something

Our brains thrive when we give it additional information to process. Something as simple as going for a drive with the family down unfamiliar roads or taking an alternative route to work can give your brain some much-needed stimulation. When I find myself stuck on a problem, I often try to take myself out of what is familiar and go somewhere new. Being in an unfamiliar setting can help you see problems and solutions in a whole new light.

Practice Yoga

Yoga can give your brain a boost while also getting you in shape. Because it combines complex movements, new movements, meditation, and breathing, it benefits our brain in ways scientists have yet to understand. If yoga isn't your thing, you might also consider Tai Chi to help you stay focused and sharpen your thinking and memory.

Learn Something New

New stimuli ALWAYS cause our brain to work harder to make sense of it. Therefore, every time we learn something new, we build our brains. If you recall, earlier in this book, we spoke about high school science and how I sucked at chemistry. Of course, it was because I had no available reference to draw on when confronted with the new material they expected me to learn. The more you can learn, the easier it makes learning in the future. That is simply because it gives you a greater base from which to compare and contrast new stimuli you are receiving with things you learned or observed previously.

IN THAT SAME WAY, if you are about to be confronted with something new to learn, you can prime your brain. This can help you keep substantially more information than you otherwise would have been able to. Here's how:

1. Before you venture into learning something new, make a list of 5-10 top-level things you already know about that subject.

2. Now take that list, and under each of those 5-10 top-level items, put down something you know about each one.

3. In your mind, try to draw a line connecting how the new subject you're about to learn pertains to each of those top-level items and the 2nd level items beneath it.

. . .

4. All done, you have now connected multiple pieces of information in your brain, and you are primed to learn something new.

Don't Use Lists

NEXT TIME you go to the grocery store, don't make a list. Force yourself to remember everything on it using one of the mnemonic devices you learned. If you are chicken, it's ok to write a list and keep it in your pocket, but don't use it. You are practicing building your memory like you would doing bicep curls at the gym. The more you force your brain to struggle, the easier and easier it becomes to remember what you need to in the future.

Be Hyper Observant

NEXT TIME you're out and about, focus on the surrounding things. How are the people dressed? What are their mannerisms like? Take notice of the environment you're in? What type of wallpaper is on the walls, and what colors do you see? Take yourself out of that comfort state of ignorant bliss and truly focus on every detail around you. Then once you leave, try to remember every single detail that you took notice of. Practice this daily, and it is one of the easiest and best ways to build your memory. Here is a game I developed to test and build my memory:

1. Pick 10 specific details to remember (color of the wallpaper, type of flooring, the person's outfit, the person's facial expression, etc.). I try to do this when I am at a store; it doesn't work at home or a place your intimately familiar with.

2. While you are in the moment, really concentrate on those details and take in every aspect of them.

3. When you make it back to your car, immediately playback all those details in your mind, try to remember how many of the 10 details you recalled. To make this both more challenging and more impactful, I try to remember everything in sequence as I recall it in my mind.

4. Repeat this activity and next time, try to recall things 10 minutes later, 30 minutes later, 3 hours later.

DOING this each day will help your observational skills and build your memory. It's one of the easiest and most powerful ways to build your memory and track how well you encode, store, and recall memory. If you can remember the details of a grocery store the next day with ease, you know that when you hyper-focus on a conversation or presentation, you can remember that later as well.

$\cdot\quad\cdot\quad\cdot$

THERE YOU HAVE a list of a few of the easier methods to strengthen that brain muscle. There are also many apps designed to help you build your attention and memory. Some such as BrainHQ or Lumosity are fun and really deliver on their promise. I recommend ditching games on your phone that do not build your brain and replace them with apps that make you think critically. That way, the next time you're stuck on the subway, instead of wasting precious minutes on nonsense, you're improving your most important muscle.

As You're Aging

FOR THOSE OF you reading this book and wondering what you can do to slow down cognitive decline as you age, I would again reference this chapter. Everything that is in this chapter will apply to you as you get older. However, it becomes less of a suggestion and more of a necessity. Keeping your senses sharp by utilizing them and continuing to learn will stimulate your brain. The biggest way to keep your wits about you and preserve your memory as you age is simply believing in your ability. If you didn't buy into the limitations and stereotypes the world put on you when you were young, why believe them now? Or perhaps you didn't always have that self-assurance, but you are also wiser when you are older. You have seen more and experienced more, and so take a

moment each day to appreciate who you are and what
you can do.

Training your brain doesn't have to be scary or difficult,
but it has to be intentional. You must force yourself to seek
ways to practice what you have learned every day.
Becoming complacent and lazy is easy to do. It's not
because you don't care or are a bad person; rather, compla-
cency results from exhaustion in body and mind. My challenge to you is to take what you learn and keep the
excitement. If you can practice just a small amount each
day by the end of a month, you will have massive
improvements in your cognition and memory. Rome
wasn't built in a day, but each day they did lay bricks.
Don't give up and stay the course, and one day your brain
will thank you!

Conclusion

 "Remembrance of things past is not necessarily the remembrance of things as they were."

— Marcel Proust

So, are you going to try it out now? You've learned all about memory, beliefs, and habits that increase your ability to remember. You know what to eat and what to avoid to make the process easier. Mnemonic devices are now your friends, and you learned my favorite, The Memory Palace. Follow the step-by-step guide on how to create a Memory Palace so you can gain the superpower of incredible memorization. You need your memory to work perfectly. It's useful for work, school, personal relationships, and personal development. Creating a Memory Palace is also helpful for when you need to have fun with your brain. Exercising your brain strengthens it and improves future performance. Create your palace and invent your world while you assist your memory to become better.

It's all on you now; you don't have any excuses not to take steps to gain better memory. Don't delay; start today on the training to take back control of your most important muscle. If you go to the gym every day and have a killer body, that's amazing. But guess what, your outward muscles will fade as you age, and you won't ever look as good in 30 years as you do today. The one thing that sticks with you and is useful at any age is a sharp mind and an excellent memory. Focus on what will matter in 3o years, and you won't ever look back with regret. I truly hope you enjoyed The Ultimate Memory Manual and become a better you because of it. Be sure to visit JONNELSEN.COM to see my other books, dedicated to helping you reach all the potential you can reach!

**If you enjoyed this book please leave an honest review.
It really does make a HUGE difference!**

~ Jon Nelsen

125

References

How to Build a Memory Palace - Memory Techniques Wiki. Artofmemory.com. (2020). Retrieved May 12 2020, from https://artofmemory.com/wiki/How_to_Build_a_Memory_Palace.

Greenwood, P.M., Baldwin, C.L., Espeseth, T., Thompson, J.C., Jiang, X., Foster, P.P. (2020). Cognitive and Brain Aging: Interventions to Promote Well-Being in Old Age. Roadmap for Interventions Preventing Cognitive Aging. ISBN: 9782889634897.

Horsley, K. (2016). Unlimited Memory: How to Use Advanced Learning Strategies to Learn Faster, Remember More, and be More Productive. TCK Publishing.

Horsley, K. (2020). How to Improve Your Memory: A Simple Memory Technique That Allows You to. TCK Publishing. Retrieved May 15 2020, from https://www.tckpublishing.com/how-to-improve-your-memory/.

Metivier, A., & Metivier, A. (2020). How to Build A Memory Palace: A Scientifically Proven Approach. Magnetic Memory Method - How to Memorize With A Memory Palace. Retrieved May 17 2020, from https://www.magneticmemorymethod.com/memory-palace/.

In Praise of Memorization: 10 Proven Brain Benefits - BestCollegesOnline.com. BestCollegesOnline.com. (2020). Retrieved May 15 2020, from https://www.bestcollegesonline.com/blog/in-praise-of-memorization-10-proven-brain-benefits/.

Higher grades and other benefits of a good memory. ABS-CBN News. (2020). Retrieved May 13 2020, from https://news.abs-cbn.com/lifestyle/05/10/12/higher-grades-and-other-benefits-good-memory.

How Important is Good Memory in Business? Illumine.-co.uk. (2020). Retrieved May 21 2020, from https://www.illumine.co.uk/2016/02/important-good-memory-business/.

Why Memory Matters For All of Us | Benefits of Having a Good Memory. Hope Grows. (2020). Retrieved May 17 2020, from https://hopegrows.net/news/why-having-a-good-memory-matters.

8 Main Causes of Forgetting. Psychology Discussion - Discuss Anything About Psychology. (2020). Retrieved May 21 2020, from https://www.psychologydiscussion.net/mind/8-main-causes-of-forgetting/2056/.

Fotuhi, M. (2003). The Memory Cure: How to Protect Your Brain Against Memory Loss and Alzheimer's. McGraw-Hill.

Howard LeWine, M. (2020). Too little sleep, and too much, affect memory - Harvard Health Blog. Harvard Health Blog. Retrieved May 21 2020, from https://www.health.harvard.edu/blog/little-sleep-much-affect-memory-201405027136.

Olin, K., Boyd, S., & Hooks, K. (2020). This is Us [Film]. Los Angeles, California; NBC Films.

Schacter, D. (2009). The seven sins of memory. W. Ross MacDonald School Resource Services Library.

"Can You Train Your Brain to Get a Photographic Memory?." 27 Feb. 2020, https://www.healthline.com/health/mental-health/how-to-get-a-photographic-memory. Accessed 26 Dec. 2020.

"What Is the Memory Capacity of the Human Brain? - Scientific ...." 1 May. 2010, https://www.scientificamerican.com/article/what-is-the-memory-capacity/. Accessed 26 Dec. 2020.

"Hyderabad kid enters Guinness Book - india - Hindustan Times." 7 Sep. 2006, https://www.hindustantimes.com/india/hyderabad-kid-enters-guinness-book/story-G4EYyOHSctytbG1z5jmUQI.html. Accessed 26 Dec. 2020.

"Good memory is 'key to happiness' - BBC News - BBC.com." 17 Sep. 2010, https://www.bbc.com/news/uk-scotland-tayside-central-11342947?SThisFB. Accessed 26 Dec. 2020.

"The effectiveness of eye–closure in repeated interviews ...." https://bpspsychub.onlinelibrary.wiley.com/doi/abs/10.1111/lcrp.12013. Accessed 26 Dec. 2020.

"Dr. Sean Lane, Louisiana State University – Liars and Lying ...." 6 Jan. 2014, https://www.wamc.org/post/dr-sean-lane-louisiana-state-university-liars-and-lying. Accessed 26 Dec. 2020.

"35 Crazy Facts about Your Memory | Best Life." 28 Jun. 2018, https://bestlifeonline.com/facts-about-memory/. Accessed 26 Dec. 2020.

"You Can Train Your Brain Just Like Any Other Muscle ...." https://integratedlistening.com/you-can-train-your-brain-just-like-any-other-muscle/. Accessed 26 Dec. 2020.

Goldstein, B. (2011). Cognitive Psychology: Connecting Mind, Research, and Everyday Experience--with coglab manual. (3rd ed.). Belmont, CA: Wadsworth.

Morris MC, Evans DA, Tangney CC, Bienias JL, Wilson RS. Fish consumption and cognitive decline with age in a large community study. Arch Neurol. 2005 Dec;62(12):1849-53. doi: 10.1001/archneur.62.12.noc50161. Epub 2005 Oct 10. PMID: 16216930.

Nehlig A. Effects of coffee/caffeine on brain health and disease: What should I tell my patients? Pract Neurol. 2016 Apr;16(2):89-95. doi: 10.1136/practneurol-2015-001162. Epub 2015 Dec 16. PMID: 26677204.

"11 Best Foods to Boost Your Brain and Memory - Healthline." 7 Jul. 2020, https://www.healthline.com/nutrition/11-brain-foods. Accessed 30 Dec. 2020.

Smells Ring Bells: How Smell Triggers Memories and Emotions. (2015, January 12). Retrieved December 31, 2020, from https://www.psychologytoday.com/us/blog/brain-babble/201501/smells-ring-bells-how-smell-triggers-memories-and-emotions

www.ingramcontent.com/pod-product-compliance
Lightning Source LLC
Chambersburg PA
CBHW031230250726
48655CB00005B/1885